ME/Chronic Fatigue Syn

A Path Back to Life

The Art of Micro-Rehab

"If you have ME/CFS then this book can help you"

STEVEN J. SOMMER MD
with **TORI SOMMER DC**
Contribution by Ruth Gador

Audiobook & eBook versions available at
drstevensommer.com

A Path Back to Life by Steven J. Sommer M.D.

Copyright © 2022 Steven J Sommer, MD. All rights reserved. Except for scholarly fair use and quotations for purposes of review, no part of this book may be reproduced without written permission of the author.

ISBN 978-0-9954345-5-4

DISCLAIMER

This book has been created to bring hope, understanding and direction to individuals (and their families and friends), facing ME/Chronic Fatigue Syndrome (ME/CFS). It is not intended in any way to replace other professional health care advice, but to support it. Readers of this publication agree that neither Dr Steven Sommer nor Tori Sommer will be held responsible or liable for damages that may be alleged or resulting, directly, or indirectly, from their use of the information shared in this publication. All external links are provided as a resource only and are not guaranteed to remain active for any length of time. Neither author can be held accountable for the information provided by or actions resulting from accessing these other resources.

To maintain anonymity, patient's names have been changed.

I am using ME/CFS as an abbreviation for and Myalgic Encephalomyelitis also known as Chronic Fatigue Syndrome, which most researchers believe to be the same disease.

ALSO BY DR STEVEN SOMMER

A Doctor's Journey Back to Health - **Print, eBook and Audiobook available at www.drstevensommer.com**

Finding Hope – Inspiring stories, Healing insights and Health Research 2017 – **book available at www.drstevensommer.com**

Restoring Balance – **meditation/relaxation-based stress management 2009- CD & Download audio recording available at www.drstevensommer.com**

Dedication

To all those affected by ME/CFS.

ACKNOWLEDGEMENTS

Thank you to all my patients and friends who shared their stories with us so that we could share them with you. I offer particular thanks to Ruth Gador for her willingness and eloquence in contrasting her experience with ME/CFS in two essays written 12 years apart and for providing the touches of violin in the audiobook. Thanks also to Rob and Rosemary Gador, Ruth's support crew.

My wife Tori for her role as a sounding board, editor, narrator and one-person cheer squad when I needed it most. Dr Denise Ruth, Dr Judy Singer, Drs Daniel and Bev Lewis, Dr Vicki Kotsirilos, Dr Joe DiStefano, Dr Sandra Palmer and Laurie Lacey for their generosity, friendship kindness, care and help in our hour of need.

The 'Powerful Poets' luncheon lines group gatherings where we shared our writing, were precious and kept me on track. Tori, Therese Van Wegen and the late Caspar von Diebitsch thank you all. A big thank you too to Dr Bambi Ward for her constructive feedback on an earlier draft and David Gallaway for proof reading.

My thanks to fellow authors Justine Day, Liz Flaherty, Margot Maurice and her partner John Gallagher for their belief in me as a writer. Margot may no longer be here, but her lessons and spirit of encouragement live on in my heart.

Thanks also to John Garrity for his education, direction and assistance in setting up a home-studio in which Tori could narrate the audiobook.

For the most part, unless published elsewhere, the names and identifying details of the patients and friends mentioned have been changed to preserve anonymity.

CONTENTS

INTRODUCTION ix
Chapter 1 An Unexpected Friendship.. 1
Chapter 2 Changing the Terrain - The Power of Lifestyle............................... 5
Chapter 3 Finding Hope – A Treatment Plan 15
Chapter 4 Integrating Complementary Therapies (CT's) 25
Chapter 5 Choice & Progress 37
Chapter 6 Reaching Out - Building Social Scaffolding 45
Chapter 7 Restorative Sleep – Reclaiming Nigh Nigh's 53
Chapter 8 Nutritional Wisdom 69
Chapter 9 Low GI Diet and mini fasts 79
Chapter 10 Pacing and the Energy Envelope 91
Chapter 11 The Art of Micro-Rehab 103
Chapter 12 Preparation for Exercise 115
Chapter 13 STOP! The Rest Activity Dance 129
Chapter 14 GO... gently! The Rest/Activity Dance..................................... 139
Chapter 15 Defuse the Loop 153
Chapter 16 Ruth circa 2022 175
Summing Up... 181
Future Research... 187
APPENDIX 1 ME/CFS Canadian Clinical Diagnostic Criteria 2003 Summary ..193
APPENDIX 2 SYMPTOM QUESTIONNAIRE 197
APPENDIX 3 Other Possible Causes (Differential Diagnosis) 199
APPENDIX 4 Whole Food Low GI Diet Suggestions 201
APPENDIX 5 Belly Breathing 205
APPENDIX 6 Meditation and Relaxation Exercises 209
Further Reading... 217
APPENDIX 7 Automatic Negative Thoughts (ANTS) and Positive
Emotional Thoughts (PETS)... 219

CONTENTS

Further Resources 225
References ME/CFS 229
About the Authors 243
Glossary of Acronyms 247

INTRODUCTION

"I was just delighted to be able to learn there were things I could do myself that could really make a difference."
THERESE

Close to two hundred and fifty thousand Australians and millions of people worldwide are impacted by ME/CFS. While diagnostic guidelines are clear (see Appendix 1) treatment guidelines are not. They're often uninspiring and unhopeful, weighed down by the need to focus on what people cannot do rather than what they can do. This tends to leave people in limbo waiting for a medical cure. This may come, but I was waiting for this cure 17 years ago. Fortunately, I found another way.[1]

My story, shared in *A Doctor's Journey Back to Health,* along with the stories you will read in this book, demonstrate there is much that can be done. Enormous benefits are possible so that the person with ME/CFS, whilst not necessarily cured, can find their world opens up in unexpected ways. How so? The devil, as they say, is in the detail, and this is the subject of this book.

A Biomedical Disease

As I've examined in my previous book, there is now consensus amongst medical scientists; the war for validity is over, i.e., we are dealing with a serious biomedical neurological disease not a psychiatric one.[2,3] Whilst the science continues to validate the reality of ME/CFS, the battle for effective biomedical treatments has barely begun. There have been shimmers of hope, like the immune modifying medication Rituximab, once touted as a possible solution but after years of research found not to be the answer.[4]

Hence, whilst not denying the possibility of curative medications being discovered, this book will focus largely on what you can do to help yourself right NOW.

Don't get me wrong, as our understanding of this disease grows it is possible a specific diagnostic test and treatment may be just around the corner, but then again, as I admitted earlier, I was waiting for this 17 years ago, and thank goodness I decided to wait no longer before doing what I could to find a way to a better life.

Hence, through applying personal and clinical experience along with extensive best-practice medical and scientific research, this book presents a framework for treatment.

N-of-1 Research

At this point in time, it is early days in terms of research into rehabilitation treatments for ME/CFS. So how can we know what to choose? N-of-1 research can help us out here.[5] This research method involves a single person - you the reader for example (n-of-1= number of people being studied = 1) - and your response to a treatment. So, for example, you could use the Appendix 2 symptom questionnaire before and after you introduce a new lifestyle measure, like for example the low GI diet I suggest in Chapter 9, then you'll have a record of how you felt before you started the new diet and then compare it to your results after completing the same questionnaire after one month on the new diet. By then you'll generally have an answer about its benefit or not. This n-of-1 research technique can be applied to any treatment you choose to test.

In terms of ME/CFS, as I've said above, lifestyle research is limited but this research technique allows you to circumvent this by doing your own. This will help you to build your own safe parameters, for say pacing homework, as you increase knowledge of yourself and your capacities.

Micro-Rehab

> "Make haste slowly."
> **AFRICAN PROVERB**

The idea of 'less is more' is relevant to a variety of areas in medicine. For example, minute doses of peanut butter are being given to young children to treat their allergy to peanuts (please don't try this at home!) by carefully desensitising their immune systems.[6] Micro-dosing with tiny doses of psychiatric medication are being trialled to improve wellbeing.[7] I posit that this 'less is more' trend is very relevant when treating ME/CFS. It is well known that smaller than usual doses of medication, especially to begin with, tend to be more beneficial for people with ME/CFS and now we can apply this same principle to physical rehab.

There is growing research demonstrating the importance and benefit of physical movement with an appropriate level of challenge in the management of all neurological disorders. For instance, there are specific exercise programs to help rehabilitate people with Parkinson's and Multiple Sclerosis.[8-12] These may not take the illnesses away but make life so much more enjoyable. How to do this safely in ME/CFS, without inducing the wrath of post-exertional malaise (PEM), is what I refer to here as Micro-Rehab, and this is the individual art that I will teach you in this book.

I developed the Micro-Rehab approach specifically for ME/CFS over time as it became apparent that the methods of rehabilitation being used for other chronic diseases would not apply or need significant modification in order to avoid PEM, particularly in the initial three to six months. Micro-Rehab is based upon increasing conscious (as opposed to anxious) self-awareness, for if you are looking through a lens of anxiety, this will disrupt your attempts at pacing appropriately and will need to be addressed. The less anxious you are the more accurately you can mindfully apply this awareness to doll out sustainable amounts of energy for your activities of daily living and individualise and build upon this via Micro-Rehab.

The Micro-Rehab approach is no quick fix. While it's true there were a handful of my patients who'd had ME/CFS for less than a year who returned to near normal health within three months when they applied this approach, these were the exceptions. Most people I saw either had ME/CFS for much longer or had a more severe version. These people would usually require many months or years of patient persistence to return their health to a place where they were able to participate more fully in life's activities again. But as I used to ask them; "Have you got something better to do?"

Is it Worth the Effort?

Until my friend and rheumatologist Dr Daniel Lewis arrived at my front door in 2004, I'd been spending money I could not really afford, on 'promising but unproven' remedies most of which did little to help. Like so many people with ME/CFS I was waiting…, waiting…, hoping that a specific treatment would emerge to at least make my life easier. No such remedy arrived.

Serendipitously, Dr Lewis and his rehab-team-leading physio and yoga teacher, Laurie Lacey, (see A Doctor's Journey back to Health Ch 15) set me on a different path from which I could find a way to extract myself from the mire I was in. It wasn't easy though; they did not have all the answers and I needed to modify their approach.

INTRODUCTION

To 'make haste slowly' was a challenge for me too, especially so until my brain-fogged head began to clear. Believe me, if a simpler treatment arises that really works, I will be the first to scream, "Take It!" and won't be offended at all if you then toss this book in the recycle bin! Then again, if the history of other neurological disorders (Parkinson's, MS, strokes etc.,) is anything to go by, the Micro-Rehab principles you will learn here, are likely to synergize with whatever other specific treatments may arise, so maybe don't toss this book out just yet!

Is it Safe?

This was a common question I got from new patients especially those who had encountered advice of caution regarding exercise from support groups. Yes! It is safe. You are the driver. Through self-awareness and biofeedback, you will establish your safe starting point and build slowly from there. This can be adapted even for people with severe cases of ME/CFS.

Once you find a safe starting point, no matter how seemingly trivial, you have a place to begin. This will be explained in detail in Chapter 12. Although it might seem tortoise-like at first, recovery of at least some of your past energies and abilities will tend to gain momentum with time, especially if you stick with it for at least 3 months. Along the way you might even pick up some unexpected additional life-skills.

My Challenge

In my clinic I applied an individualized, rather than generic approach with each person I saw. But could I translate this approach for the many in compiling this book? This was my challenge. Like the illness itself, which can be so infuriating, there were times when trying to pull this all together in a way that was accessible and hopefully interesting to you the reader, almost led me to scream, "TOO HARD!" and lob the keyboard out the window.

Then, after taking a break and recalling the memory of what it meant to me to have some direction to apply myself to in 2004, (see A Doctor's Journey Back to Health Ch 15), I would reassure my innocent keyboard of my good intentions and go again. To my joy, over time, it allowed me to distill my knowledge in a way that was even clearer than I'd been able to do in my Practice years.

We will begin and end the book with Ruth Gador's story, described in her words in two essays. Ruth first consulted with me with ME/CFS at the age of 18 in 2008. These two essays contrast her experience of life then and now, two points in time, 12 years apart.

We'll then look at the hidden power of lifestyle in treating disease by changing our *'milieu intérieur' or terrain*. Hope, intuition, Complementary Therapies and typical patterns of progress will all be touched upon before, ultimately, we review in depth each of eight-steps in a rehabilitation approach to ME/CFS including the critical Micro-Rehab component.

Make haste slowly; take your time. Assess and/or intuit which are the most relevant lessons for you then apply them to your situation. May they change your life's trajectory for the good.

Dr Steven Sommer MBBS, FRACGP
Geelong February, 2022

Chapter 1
AN UNEXPECTED FRIENDSHIP
RUTH GADOR CIRCA 2008

Let's begin with an essay written by one of my patients, Ruth, a bright 31-year-old violin teacher and musician. Upon completion of her VCE (high school), Ruth had been accepted into studying music at Melbourne University. She decided to take a gap year before commencing. It was during this fateful year, at the age of 18, following a series of viral illnesses coupled with a stressful employment situation, that she developed ME/CFS. Her experience of ME/CFS included severe Postural Orthostatic Tachycardia Syndrome (POTS). This meant that when I first consulted with Ruth, POTS had left her unable to sit upright for more than 10 minutes before needing to lie down or risk fainting due to falling blood pressure. Her essay, An Unexpected Friendship (below) was first published in Emerge magazine, the quarterly Journal of ME/CFS Australia (VicTasNT).[1] In her words…

An Unexpected Friendship by Ruth Gador

Five years ago, I contracted Chronic Fatigue Syndrome. I would like to share with you all a rather unusual friendship, which has evolved over this period of time. I would never in my wildest dreams have expected something so joyful to come out of being socially isolated and housebound. I hope you can appreciate the humor of it, and may it bring a smile to your face.

For me, it represents the small, simple pleasures in life that I have learnt to appreciate, value and cherish since becoming so ill.

So, with no further ado, I shall begin.

I have a little dog called Jaco. He's a black and white foxy cross with a Jack Russell, and he is absolutely gorgeous (although I do admit I am rather biased!) I don't know how I would have survived without him these past five years. I know that for many of you reading this who have pets, you will understand my attachment.

When I was initially diagnosed, I was constantly dizzy and unable to walk very far without aid. That first winter Jaco spent many days curled up with me at the foot of the couch, snuggled against my feet and cushioned in my warm, green blanket. He was such a comfort to me.

And there he would stay…except for the same time each day, when he would suddenly go crazy, barking like mad. He'd rush to the door in a frenzy to get out. I'd hear him howling fit to burst for two minutes or so. And then, as suddenly as it began, he would come back inside, snuggle right back down against my feet, and go to sleep again.

Now, it didn't take long for my curiosity to become aroused. What on earth was happening each day? Who, or what, was so important for Jaco to see?

Well, the next day I waited for the scheduled time. I was prepared and had saved up enough energy that morning to make it to the front door off the couch at said time. To my utter astonishment, coming down the street was a big, big man with a fat, waddling black and white Dalmatian by his side. Jaco sprang out to greet them, barking fit to burst. However, what eventuated next perplexed me further…as the man seemed to know *Jaco's name!* He called out to him jovially, started talking to him, laughing with him, and then proceeded to tell him off for his rude, barking behavior. *His* dog, might I add, was impeccably well behaved during this entire episode, he didn't even blink an eyelid at the annoying little dog trying to terrorize him through the fence.

Well, from that day on, this interaction was something that I gleefully looked forward to every morning. Come rain or shine, it was a constant

CHAPTER I AN UNEXPECTED FRIENDSHIP

that I could rely on, and that I could *enjoy*, no matter how terrible I felt. I'd wait for the time, and sure enough a chuckle would escape from my lips and a big grin would spread over my face as I peeped through the window, watching for *Mr. Man*; a name I quickly coined for this strange gentleman (to whose real name I had utterly no idea). Every now and then I'd go outside too, if I was feeling strong enough. Over time, we slowly got to the point where we both felt the bonds of familiarity emerge, and we managed a small wave to each other; never a word though, mind you. No, this man, *Mr. Man,* was one of those rare species of men that we like to call *'dog people.'* But that didn't trouble me. After all, the way I saw it, the less talking I had to do, the better.

That year, for the first time in the history of Jaco's life, he received a Christmas card. It was entitled 'Jaco and Family.' I froze. 'It couldn't be,' I thought, and then proceeded to open the envelope with trembling fingers.

'Yes, it could!'

Written on a beautiful RSPCA doggie card was a heartfelt message of thanks and gratitude to Jaco and his owners. That is possibly the most exciting Christmas card I have ever received. And best of all...*I finally found out Mr. Man's real name!*

It still amazes me to this day that something so...normal could become a source of such great amusement.

We'll return to Ruth's story in Chapter 16.

Chapter 2
CHANGING THE TERRAIN - THE POWER OF LIFESTYLE

> *"Bernard was right, the terrain is everything...*
> *the microbe nothing."*
> **LOUIS PASTEUR 1822-1895**

An Old Debate

The above quote, attributed on his deathbed to the scientist widely acknowledged as the founder of microbiology, Louis Pasteur, refers to Claude Bernard another prominent French medical scientist (physiologist) of that time.[1] While there is a great deal of controversy over this quote's attribution to Pasteur, for our purposes it neatly delineates two ways in which we can tackle ME/CFS.

Homeostasis - The Wisdom of the Body

While chemist Pasteur is well known and renowned for his discoveries of the principles of vaccination, microbial fermentation, and pasteurization, less well known is fellow scientist, Bernard. Claude Bernard is also considered to be one of the 'greatest of all men of science.'[2] His accomplishments include being one of the first to suggest the use of a blinded experiment to ensure the objectivity of scientific observations. He also originated the term *milieu intérieur*, or terrain, and a process that became known as 'homeostasis,' a term Harvard physiology professor Walter Cannon went on to popularly coin in his 1932 book, *The Wisdom of the Body*.[3]

If one recognises 'the wisdom of the body' then it becomes clear that the food we eat, the air we breathe, the exercise we choose, the stress we feel, the rest and sleep we get all interact and can influence the body's inbuilt self-healing systems. Bernard believed, in contrast to Pasteur's famous discovery of the germ theory of disease, that the state of health of the body and its capacity to repel disease was more important than the microbe attacking it. This is where homeostasis comes in.

Homeostasis is the body's ability to maintain a finely tuned equilibrium in many areas of its function by self-monitoring and regulating its internal environment in response to changes in the external environment. Examples include maintaining an appropriate body temperature, pH (acid-base balance), immune defences, respiratory (breathing) rate, heart rate and blood pressure.

Because pasteurization, immunization, sterilization and antibiotics have been so effective at preventing and treating illnesses, factors that enhance homeostasis like, fresh air, a healthy diet, laughter, a walk in nature, good company, better sleep etc., tend not to be considered as so important a medicine anymore. Yet, we now know that *both* the microbe *and* the terrain (intérieur milieu) are important in keeping us healthy or making us sick.

COVID 19

A modern-day example is COVID 19. We know the virus causing it is SARS-CoV-2 and that it is transmissible through fine droplet spread in the air and on surfaces. This knowledge of the microbe has allowed us to use ways to avoid it (e.g., masks and social distancing) as well as to develop effective vaccines and hopefully soon specific antiviral treatments.

Less well known is that people with low vitamin D levels (often from a lack of sunlight exposure) are more susceptible to catching COVID[4] as are people with diabetes and obesity.

Those with obesity, defined as having a Body Mass Index (BMI) of more than 30 compared to those with a BMI < 30, have a risk of ending up in hospital with Covid-19 that increases by 113%; of needing intensive care by 74%, and of dying of the virus by 48%.[5]

Clearly the terrain the virus finds itself in is very important.

Further Evidence of the Importance of Terrain

Here is a self-explanatory abstract from research published in the journal, *Science, back in 1984:*

> "Records on recovery after cholecystectomy (gallbladder removal surgery) of patients in a suburban Pennsylvania hospital between 1972 and 1981 were examined to determine whether assignment to a room with a window view of a natural setting might have restorative influences. Twenty-three surgical patients assigned to rooms with windows looking out on a natural scene had shorter postoperative hospital stays, received fewer negative evaluative comments in nurses' notes, and took fewer potent analgesics (painkillers) than 23 matched patients in similar rooms with windows facing a brick building wall."[6]

Here is another abstract from research published in 1998:

> "We report a natural experiment that took place in a cardiac intensive care unit (CICU). The 628 subjects were patients admitted directly to the CICU with a first attack of myocardial infarction (MI) - i.e., heart attack. Outcomes of those treated in sunny rooms and those treated in dull rooms were retrospectively compared for fatal outcomes and for length of stay in the CICU.

Patients stayed a shorter time in the sunny rooms, but the significant difference was confined to women (2.3 days in sunny rooms, 3.3 days in dull rooms). Mortality in both sexes was **consistently higher in dull rooms** *(39/335 dull, 21/293 sunny). We conclude that illumination may be relevant to outcome in MI, and that this natural experiment merits replication.[7]"*

The same researchers had found profound benefits for depressed patients of a sunlit room compared with a dull room on their psychiatric ward - "*Those in sunny rooms had an* **average stay of 16.9 days compared to 19.5 days** *for those in dull rooms, a difference of 2.6 days (15%): P < 0.05.*"[8]

How Does All This Relate to ME/CFS?

While research continues, we have yet to find a cause (e.g., a microbe, toxin or specific autoimmune reaction) for ME/CFS and hence no specific treatments, such as antibiotics or autoimmune medication to treat it. But due to our understanding of homeostasis, we need not feel helpless in the face of this, because while waiting for the cure we can alter the terrain, that is, the environment which can either improve ME/CFS (e.g., exposing ourselves to fresh air and natural light, by improving diet, sleep patterns, strengthening muscles etc.) or worsen it (e.g., through mostly being in a dull airless rooms, a poor diet, poor sleep patterns, deconditioning by avoiding all exercise etc.).

Epigenetics and Neuroplasticity

Yet, I hear you ask, how can these, seemingly simple lifestyle measures (referred by some doctors as 'general measures' – as opposed to specific treatments like drugs or surgery) help us recover from such a serious neurological disease like ME/CFS?

While Pasteur and Bernard would no doubt be gob smacked at the advancement of modern medical science, perhaps we are rediscovering what they (or certainly Bernard) knew, that the terrain, some of which we can influence, can **treat** disease. In my previous book, *A Doctor's Journey Back to Health – Chapter 14 Epigenetic Switches,* we have a clue as to how this might occur. We now know genes, which carry the codes that literally build our bodies, can be switched on or off depending on the environment they find themselves in. When combined with our understanding of neuroplasticity in which new connections literally can grow in our brains in response to repeated inputs, it shows us just how important our choices and behaviors can be.

Dr Ornish's Research

In my book, *Finding Hope,* I touched on some of the work and research published by cardiologist Dr Dean Ornish and colleagues. In 1990 when his first ground-breaking research paper in *The Lancet*[9] demonstrated that ischaemic heart disease could be reversed with lifestyle change alone i.e., given the right terrain the body could unplug cholesterol plaques on its own without medication or invasive medical or surgical interventions. This was considered impossible by most cardiologists (heart specialists) at that time.

I was working as a senior lecturer in the Department of General Practice at Monash University Medical School and I became inspired by the potential this implied for all of us. Could other serious diseases have this possibility too? Could we actually treat our illnesses with specific lifestyle change not just prevent them with lifestyle as I'd been taught?[10-13]

Dr Ornish's research team then looked at whether lifestyle change might reverse the course of early prostate cancer through epigenetic mechanisms. Five-year follow up research showed this to be true, with corresponding alterations in beneficial gene expression and survival. Backing up the importance of Bernard's insight, those who committed themselves to the lifestyle change the most did the best.[14-18]

While I'm unaware of any such holistic lifestyle-based research into ME/CFS, research into a neuro-immune disorder with some similarity to ME/CFS, Multiple Sclerosis (MS), provides encouraging evidence that people with MS can positively affect the course of their illness over at least a 5-year period by changing their lifestyle.[19-23]

There is also consistent research into Parkinson's disease demonstrating significant reductions in symptoms, the slowing down of progression and in some cases disease reversal through regular appropriate exercise.[24]

As the growing body of research under the banner of Lifestyle Medicine and Mind-body Medicine increases, there is a recognition that one size does **not** fit all. Different illnesses and individuals within the same illness-grouping may need different individualized lifestyle-treatments.[25] This challenges researchers and clinicians to come up with more flexible protocols and research methodologies. As I said at the end of Chapter 14 in *A Doctor's Journey Back to Health*, I don't believe all aspects of the Ornish Lifestyle program to be suitable for people with ME/CFS. The reasons for this will become obvious in the chapters that follow as we hone-in on some of the specific lifestyle approaches that ARE suitable for treating ME/CFS.

The Magic of Synergy

In the early 90's the Anti-Cancer Council employed me to present 'How to Quit Smoking' educational talks to groups of smokers attempting to quit. Many were unfamiliar with the concept of synergy. Simply put, for many illnesses, like lung cancer and cardiovascular disease, the risk multiplies rather than just adds with each extra risk factor you have. For example, high blood pressure and high cholesterol are relatively minor risk factors for cardiovascular disease on their own but multiply in their danger if they occur together.[26]

Asbestos exposure increases your risk of developing lung cancer by five times, but if you have asbestos exposure and are a smoker, your risk multiplies to 28 times higher than average![27,28] That's synergy but not the sort of synergy you want!

The magic here is that synergy can also work the other way i.e., in a self-healing way too. For instance, if you stop smoking completely, you can return your lung cancer risk to that of a non-smoker in just 10 years. The body literally spring cleans the lungs. But as Dr Ornish demonstrated for cardiovascular disease and prostate cancer, if you adopt a wholistic lifestyle program as well as stop smoking, you can reverse some already established disease, including diseases like prostate cancer and Type 2 Diabetes. What about ME/CFS?

N-of-1 Research

I covered some of this in the *Introduction* but it is worth repeating here. At this point in time it is early days in terms of research into lifestyle treatments and ME/CFS, so how can we know what to choose? N-of-1 research can help us out here.[29] This research method involves a single person (n-of-1) and their response to a treatment.

For example, if you introduce a lifestyle measure, like say the low GI diet I suggest in Chapter 9, **note how you feel before you start the new diet and then after one month** on the new diet (using the **Appendix 2 symptom questionnaire before and after**). Then you return to your previous diet, note how you feel on this after one more month (fill in Appendix 2 questionnaire again), then repeat the low GI diet for another month before completing the questionnaire for a fourth time. You'll generally be able to notice which, if any of these two diets makes you feel better, worse or no different. This n-of-1 research technique can be applied to any lifestyle change (or other treatments for that matter) you choose to test.

In terms of ME/CFS, as I've said above, lifestyle research is limited but n-of-1-research technique allows you to circumvent this by doing your own. As I've noted above, we can also take heart from research that is mounting about the positive effects of lifestyle change on other neurological diseases such as Parkinson's Disease and MS. So, how can we use this knowledge to create positive synergy for managing ME/CFS?

Changing the Terrain in ME/CFS

If you have read the Introduction and my previous books you'll realize that both my interest as a medical doctor and lecturer at Monash Medical School and my own experience as a patient with ME/CFS, taught me the healing potential of lifestyle change and mind-body medicine. Helping people with ME/CFS to experience this, as I did in my clinic, became my passion. Seeing it work for many is in large part why I've written this book.

So, whilst I undertook some postgraduate training in Integrative/Functional/Complementary medicine, and I include a chapter on this area in this book (Chapter 4), I soon realized that to maximize health and overcome chronic diseases like ME/CFS, a focus on pacing and appropriate lifestyle change would need to be a major one, not just a token one at the end of a consultation. Hence, I undertook further training in health coaching and counselling, prescribed medication minimally, if at all, and involved a multidisciplinary team in which the person with ME/CFS was front and center, growing in self-awareness and confidence in reading their body. The patient's regular GP would be kept in the loop and if medication were needed, they would often be the one asked to prescribe this.

CHAPTER 2 CHANGING THE TERRAIN - THE POWER OF LIFESTYLE

Much as Diabetes Mellitus is now seen as a multifaceted disease requiring a multidisciplinary approach, so too I believe is ME/CFS. When a patient of mine, Katie, (you'll read Katie's story in Chapter 14), was referred to me by her GP, a well-respected integrative medicine doc in this region, I referred her on to the Austin Hospital's multidisciplinary inpatient program. After just four weeks as an inpatient in their ME/CFS program, he and I were stunned by her improvement. He rang me and told me that after 10 years of applying an Integrative medicine approach to ME/CFS, he believed that the rehab lifestyle approach I was assisting Katie with was the current best practice, in his view, in ME/CFS treatment.

I'm not telling you this to blow my own trumpet, nor do I believe it to necessarily be the main deal for *all* people with ME/CFS. In fact, in Katie's situation the Austin's rehab team were the keys here. My role was simply to anchor the strategies they'd taught her. What it does demonstrate is just how effective Bernard's terrain restoration idea CAN be for at least some people with ME/CFS.

Regardless of the other treatments you might try, appropriate lifestyle change can synergize with these to improve on your results. In the rest of this book we will examine how you can choose and integrate some of the safe effective terrain changing measures to impact your ME/CFS that have worked for me and many others with ME/CFS.

Chapter 2
Key Points

- ✓ Louis Pasteur and Claude Bernard were both great men of science in 19th century France.
- ✓ This book utilizes Bernard's concept of the *milieu intérieur* or terrain, better known today as homeostasis or wisdom of the body to tackle ME/CFS.
- ✓ Lifestyle change can both prevent and treat most disease.
- ✓ This ability to alter the course and treat disease using appropriate lifestyle change has been shown to work for cardiovascular disease, Diabetes Mellitus, prostate cancer, Parkinson's disease and Multiple Sclerosis.
- ✓ N-of-1 research allows the person with ME/CFS to more accurately choose their treatments.
- ✓ We will explore how you can improve your ME/CFS disease with ME/CFS specific lifestyle choices and mind body techniques in upcoming chapters.

Chapter 3
FINDING HOPE – A TREATMENT PLAN

"... Approaching adversity with a positive attitude at least gives you a chance of success. Approaching it with a defeatist attitude predestines the outcome."
DR BELINDA KIELY, ONCOLOGIST

The first step in treatment is to never give up hope. If anyone tells you or you hear someone say, "this is incurable and there is nothing more that can be done for you," I want you to say, at the very least internally, "Rubbish!" In my book *Finding Hope*,[1] I share numerous stories of people I have known or treated with a wide variety of medical conditions, including the Big 'C' (cancer), in which they were told exactly this, and yet they are well today, having defied the odds.

As regards ME/CFS, you will read in the following chapters about many others who've defied the gloom and doom that surrounds this diagnosis. As I've said in the previous chapter, even if there isn't a **specific** medication, herb or supplement that will miraculously return you to full health yet, and who's to say it won't be discovered soon, there are many things that can improve the '**terrain**,' unleashing your self-healing systems with often surprising benefits.

Much of the rest of this book will be devoted to sharing what I've learnt regarding the ME/CFS-specific strategies that can help you to maximize your 'terrain.'

A Caution

Be aware that people who claim to recover from ME/CFS and write books or talk about it, will often put their recovery down to 'one thing' in particular. In some situations, this may be true, but many times, this 'one thing' is simply the last piece in a complex jigsaw that has allowed everything else to click into place. They may not realize that if they had not already built up their health fundamentals through placing all the other jigsaw pieces correctly, they may not have recovered with this 'one' last piece.

In this situation you may be disappointed if you try the 'one thing' and it doesn't work for you. This can even leave you feeling inadequate; you may even fall into despair. There is only one thing to say to this too, "Rubbish!" Your own life-restoration journey is likely to be very different to theirs.

Hope - Lessons from those who have recovered

In order to maintain a positive rather than defeatist attitude, so critical as Dr Kiely suggests (see quote above), I believe it is important to seek out positive stories, like the ones being shared in this book. As long as you recognize each journey will have different nuances to yours and may have needed a different approach, they can stimulate possibilities, instill hope and help to keep our collective chins up.

Unfortunately, too many medical professionals still minimize the value of such stories using the words, 'just an anecdote' or 'not evidence based' that can deflate the inspiration and devalue the bravery that these people display for us. I recall reading footballer Alastair Lynch's ME/CFS experience (see Ch 12) which ultimately led to a recovery that allowed him to play in three AFL (Australian Rules Football) premiership teams. I was at a low point at that time and reading his book about his struggles and ultimate success was literally a lifeline for me, a clarion call to battle on.[2]

CHAPTER 3 FINDING HOPE – A TREATMENT PLAN

N-of-1 Research

We touched on this earlier; there is fortunately an increasing respect in the medical scientific community for n-of-1 research.[3] In this research it is being recognized that more in depth analysis of a single person's (n) response to treatments (of-1) can provide important clues for others and for wider trials. In the next chapter I'll review again how to become your own n-of-1 researcher.

Instinct

As you increase your self-awareness, you'll find certain stories jump off the page as the one's most relevant to your situation.

As an example, in researching for this book, I came across *Recovery from CFS - 50 personal stories*,[4] a compilation book by Alexandra Barton. It became clear there were some stories that correlated with my own and some of my patients and others less so, yet the courage they all displayed was uplifting.

Sifting through the pages, there were a few keys that reversed the illness trajectory of these 50 people with ME/CFS. As I've suggested, different keys worked for different people and we do not yet have an accurate way of predicting which of these keys will work best for everyone. Hence my recommendation to use a holistic multipronged approach to restoring your terrain. As I said above, some people will attribute their recovery to 'one thing,' not realizing or minimizing the importance of the rest of the jigsaw they've already attended to. I found the stories in Alexandra's book inspiring and hopeful. Let me outline some of the recovery keys shared by the individuals in their stories from *Recovery from CFS - 50 Personal stories*:

1. Diet – most commonly a low Glycemic Index (GI) diet that essentially cuts out all 'whites;' white bread, white rice, potatoes, white flour and sugar (See Chapter 9).

2. Pacing.
3. Restoring better sleep.
4. Mind-body therapies (we'll explore these in Ch 13-15).
5. Integrative or Functional Medicine.
6. Naturopathic approaches.
7. Appropriate exercise e.g., strength work and gentle stretching.

What was also clear from Alexandra's compilation, though not overtly spelt out, was that the chances of recovery were enhanced with adequate social support and a level of self-discipline, determination and persistence.

Find an Understanding Medical Practitioner

Finding an understanding medical practitioner knowledgeable about ME/CFS is not always easy. It has been estimated that up to 80% of people with ME/CFS are undiagnosed and miss out on appropriate treatment[5,6] ME/CFS support groups may be able to direct you here, or alternatively word-of-mouth may lead you. And if your doc does not leave you feeling like you can work with them on this, then ask for a referral or try elsewhere.

A suitable doctor can confirm the diagnosis, exclude other diagnoses, manage symptoms appropriately and direct you to other health practitioners if necessary. In addition, they can monitor progress and deal with any other secondary medical problems that may arise. They can also be of assistance to your carer if you have one.

Importantly, this book can help you and your carer to build your understanding of what's going on as well as help you to educate those around you, to build a platform of support for your shot at life-restoration. And if your doctor is open but not familiar with ME/

CHAPTER 3 FINDING HOPE – A TREATMENT PLAN

CFS they may wish to read this book which will direct them to the information they will need in order to assist you.

My Initial Consultations for People with ME/CFS

When people were referred to my clinic with a preliminary diagnosis of ME/CFS, I would start by sending them some homework. Before they came, they would be asked to write a one or two-page summary of their experience of their illness including what treatments they had tried, what helped and what did not. They would also fill in a questionnaire in which they would rate their symptoms (see Appendix 2). This questionnaire is in line with the Canadian Diagnostic Clinical Criteria - CDCC - Appendix 1, rating symptoms between one and five, one being mild and five severe. This would help us to prioritize which symptoms to work on first.

At the first visit I would review their essay and questionnaire, take a thorough history and examine them. In this exam I would include a NASA Lean Test (see *A Doctor's Journey Back to Health Ch 3*) to detect low blood pressure issues such as Neurally Mediated Hypotension (NMH), which would often have a delayed onset of 5 to 10 minutes and/or Postural Orthostatic Tachycardia Syndrome, POTS. For example, in Ruth's case (see Chapter 1), she had evidence of POTS, i.e., her blood pressure would fall while her heart rate would rise as she remained upright. This happened whenever she stood or even sat up from lying. Within 10 minutes she would feel weaker and very fatigued and would need to lay flat again, lest she faint.

After the history and examination were completed, I would order blood and/or other tests to exclude other causes, as indicated, if this had not been done already (see Appendix 3).

To confirm the diagnosis, all of this would be carefully checked off against the CDCC assessment criteria (see Appendix 1).

An ME/CFS diagnosis was established only after rigorously excluding other possibilities. As a GP practicing in this field it was vital I maintained an awareness with each and every person that the diagnosis might need to be reconsidered should new symptoms arise or the condition worsen.

Once I was confident that ME/CFS was the appropriate diagnosis, I would explain what this meant to the person, validating the reality of their real physical neurological illness and how this tied together their experience of so many wretched symptoms. This validation and explanation of their experience would often bring great relief; they were **not** going crazy!

The next step was to educate and establish, as best as possible, strong social supports, via sympathetic family or friends and/or via an ME/CFS support group. If necessary, and with the permission of the person with ME/CFS, I would also consult with their main caregivers to explain the condition as I did with Caitlin's husband. You'll meet Caitlin in Chapter 6. Where relevant, letters were written for workplace, schools or universities. Income protection insurance and/or social security issues often needed to be addressed also.

With a platform of support in train, I would explain that there was no specific magic bullet, pharmaceutical or natural therapy to treat ME/CFS, but if approached with care there were many things that could help the body and mind to heal.

I would then introduce an overview of the strategy we would be working on. With the jigsaw analogy in mind, we would look at how to enhance the terrain with the four self-management fundamentals for improving any chronic illness (see Table 1) plus the four specific ME/CFS self-management measures (see Table 2).

All eight of these measures would need to be tailored to the individual's situation. The order in which we would explore each of these components was modified depending on what people had already tried, their most troubling symptoms and instinctively what we felt it best to begin with.

Social Support	Pacing
Restorative Sleep	Micro-Rehab
Nourishing Diet	Mind-body therapies
Movement	Restoring body-mind trust
Table 1. FUNDAMENTAL 4 – ME/CFS (Relevant for all Chronic Illnesses)	**Table 2. ME/CFS SPECIFIC 4 Strategies**

The above terrain measures can enhance any other treatments you may be having.

Sleep first?

Restorative sleep management was often a first point of call as it has become apparent that sleep apnea is occurring as a secondary problem in more than 50% of people with excessive daytime sleeping and ME/CFS (See Ch 7)![7] It's thought to be due to muscle deconditioning (from inactivity) making the airway floppier so that it partially closes overnight. In some it may even be the whole problem as it can mimic ME/CFS in many ways. One of my patients who had a provisional diagnosis of ME/CFS had a sleep study and ended up being diagnosed with narcolepsy. Sleep apnea is not the only type of sleep disorder that can mimic ME/CFS (See Chapter 7).

Other Issues

Coexisting anxiety and depression are common with ME/CFS. I found anxiety to be much more prevalent than depression in the people with ME/CFS that consulted with me. This is not surprising given the research demonstrating inflammation in the brainstem where our survival fight/flight response is located (see *A Doctor's Journey Back to Health* Ch 5). There are many effective non-pharmaceutical ways to settle anxiety and we'll look at some of these in Chapter 13 to 15. The Rest/Activity Dance & Defusing the Loop.

Sensitivities

People affected by ME/CFS are generally very sensitive to medication and herbal treatments, not to mention noise, strong fragrances, visual and auditory over-stimulation and emotional stress. So, with most medication or supplements prescribed for your ME/CFS symptoms it is advisable to start at a quarter or less of the usual dose and build slowly over weeks.[8] Your benefit may come at a lower dose than the average person and that would be the dose to stop at. A caveat here; if you have a serious infection like pneumonia or septicemia that requires high doses of antibiotics then the full recommended dose will be necessary.

There are a range of medications that doctors can prescribe that may help ease some of the symptoms, such as pain, mood or sleep disorders; you may wish to explore these with a doctor familiar with ME/CFS. Some trial and error in finding the right medication(s) and/or herb(s) and supplements, along with the appropriate dosage for you is inevitably going to be involved in this process. Also, be aware of your sensitivity when coming off prescription medication, such as anti-depressants. You will often need to accomplish this very slowly.

Some of my patients, like Ruth, also experienced multiple chemical sensitivities in which strong odors, like oil paints for instance, would aggravate symptoms. Others, including myself, would find electromagnetic frequencies from devices like TV's, mobile phones, iPads or PC's would be aggravators, as too would be a very noisy environment (noise cancelling headphones can be useful). Together with my patient, we would consider strategies for avoiding or minimizing exposure until they felt ready for re-challenging.

Orthostatic Intolerance

Orthostatic intolerance (OI) refers to a fall in blood pressure when standing or in some people even just sitting upright. It can be very debilitating and can cause one to feel dizzy, fatigued, light-headed, palpitations, sore legs or faint and reduce cognitive ability. See: _https://www.dysautonomiainternational.org/pdf/RoweOIsummary.pdf_ It occurs in 95% of people with ME/CFS and is caused by a malfunctioning autonomic nervous system.[9] This can manifest as Neurally Mediated Hypotension, Postural Orthostatic Tachycardia Syndrome (POTS) and Chronotropic Intolerance (CI).

My personal experience with OI was that I struggled to stand still for more than a few minutes due to sore calves and dizziness. This was quickly relieved by sitting or lying down with my legs elevated on a cushion. Some people with ME/CFS also experience subtler symptoms, such as feeling sick, nauseous, tired, or confused during periods of sitting upright or standing still. It is sometimes misinterpreted as anxiety, but this can easily be sorted out with specific blood pressure testing as outlined in my previous book, A Doctor's Journey Back to Health.

It is important to manage this as best you can in order to be able to both feel better and to benefit from the other techniques I will teach you. I have listed potential treatments to consider as outlined by Bateman et al in the Mayo Clinic Proceedings August 25, 2021.[10]

- Hydrate well. Salt and water loading, electrolyte drinks (ask your pharmacist). Keep a bottle or glass of water nearby and sip frequently.
- Compression stockings or flight socks
- Positional changes; avoid prolonged sitting or standing
- Consistent individually tailored exercise at a level that avoids triggering PEM. HOW TO DO THIS? A way to do this is the subject of the final third of this book.
- Medications: Fludrocortisone, low-dose beta blockers, alpha-adrenergic agonists, pyridostigmine, desmopressin, ivabradine
- Intravenous saline

Chapter 3
Key Points

- ✓ Many people have restored much of their lives after ME/CFS. Find hope through positive stories.
- ✓ There are things we can learn from the approach taken by these individuals, even if our road is different to theirs. Beneficially, you can let their courage and determination to not give up inspire you to do the same.
- ✓ N-of-1 research is gaining respect and can build self-awareness and provide guidance.
- ✓ There are no specific treatments as yet for ME/CFS. The approach outlined in Tables 1 and 2 above brings about improvement by focusing on the 'terrain' (see Ch 2), utilizing a carefully individualized holistic approach. Do not underestimate how powerful this can be.
- ✓ As your self-awareness and understanding of ME/CFS grow you will realize how important each of these 8 keys is.
- ✓ Each of these 8 key measures can enhance other treatments you may be having.
- ✓ Specific suggestions for dealing with sensitivities and orthostatic intolerance end this chapter.

Chapter 4

INTEGRATING COMPLEMENTARY THERAPIES (CT'S)

"Healing is not a competition."
DR HUNTER 'PATCH' ADAMS.

Every person with ME/CFS I consulted with was using at least one complementary therapy (CT) in their attempt to get well. Many of these CT's, including ones I utilized myself, promised and cost plenty (who doesn't want a quick fix!), yet rarely delivered the life-restoring level of improvement I witnessed with Micro-rehab, the path back to life this book is exploring.

Still, I tended to see people with ME/CFS who'd tried CT's and were looking for a different approach. Anyway, this could mean I'd developed a biased view, as those people who'd had excellent responses to CT's would not have sought my help.

I must acknowledge also that there were CT's that did help me and others with ME/CFS I saw, and whilst not curative, they alleviated symptoms enough to allow a crack at rehabilitation possible. So, before I go into the rehab side of things we outlined in the previous chapter, let's check out what assistance Complementary Therapies (CTs) can provide in ME/CFS.

CT Research

What does the research show in regard to ME/CFS and complementary therapies (CTs) generally? A review paper concluded there was a lack of quality and size of research so that no conclusions could be drawn. This deficiency in research continues to limit this area. However, the authors of the review paper did qualify this with the following statement: "acupuncture and several types of meditative practice show the most promise for future scientific investigation. Likewise, magnesium, L-carnitine, (D Ribose – my addition), and S-adenosylmethionine are nonpharmacological supplements with the most potential for further research. Individualized treatment plans that involve several pharmacological agents and natural remedies appear promising as well."[1] In other words, there are promising areas of research, just not enough of it to draw definitive conclusions yet.

Budget your Dose

Another important consideration for people with ME/CFS I mentioned earlier, is that less is often more. As with medical drugs the smallest therapeutic dose is often preferable and likely to benefit the most. This is especially so with herbal remedies. Beware also of taking too many supplements at once for the same reason. People with ME/CFS tend to be sensitive responders and CT's can have side-effects. They can interact with medications too, so my advice is to **check with your doctor or pharmacist** before you trial a CT to make sure it's safe to do so and if so, start with a tiny dose and build slowly.

Another important consideration is **cost**; decide how much money you are willing to spend, understanding all the costs involved including ongoing testing and supplement costs if relevant. Be honest with yourself and your practitioner if financial stress is a real issue and budget and choose accordingly. One of the big advantages of a Rehab approach is it costs little and is self-directed.

Now, let's explore some specific CT examples.

Body and Energy Work

I start with this example first as it is, I believe, one of the most underrated of complementary therapies. Many of my patients obtained significant relief from their painful musculoskeletal symptoms and enhanced their well-being by regularly attending a bodyworker, such as an osteopath, chiropractor, Traditional Chinese Medicine (TCM) practitioner, Shiatsu practitioner or massage therapist.

Most people I saw with ME/CFS found gentle approaches to be the most beneficial. The less is more philosophy applied here too. Hence, practitioners experienced with utilizing techniques such as cranial work, craniosacral balancing, Japanese acupuncture, Moxa, Bowen massage and hands on or hands-off energy work (e.g., Reiki), tended to be chosen and persisted with the most, but once again, with a little trial and error and your intuition you'll find your way.

These methods can relieve pain and improve overall energy and mood, especially if combined with personal homework like daily stretching (e.g., yoga or physio-directed stretches), deep breathing, mindfulness and meditation.

Flower Essences

Flower essences, such as Bach Flower Remedies (e.g., Rescue Remedy found in most chemists) or Australian Bush Flower Remedies can be very helpful for easing emotional pain. With the assistance of a naturopath familiar with these remedies, they are generally selected intuitively and administered by a dropper or sprayer onto the tongue. At difficult times over my eleven year ME/CFS journey I found these remedies to be very soothing and helpful.

Healing Sounds

Soothing music such as harp music or crystal bowls can both relax and energise. There are music therapists who can assist with suggestions suitable for your current situation. Ruth, whom we met in Chapter 1 and will meet again in Chapter 16, had this to say about her experience. "In recent months, I have discovered spiritual sound healing to be a really profound way of bringing me back into balance. The sound encourages me to let go of difficult emotions and foster a deep sense of internal peace. It creates a safety net around my body and helps me to be in touch with my true emotions. Once again, I'm astounded at the power of music and sound, and the continual impact that it has in my life."

Medicinal Cannabis

Medicinal cannabis, derived from the hemp family of plants is another underrated CT. There are many different types of hemp plant; some provide excellent textile material for making clothing and rope, others have been utilized recreationally (e.g., marijuana smoking) and I certainly don't recommend this, not only is it illegal and bad for your lungs, but it carries a risk of triggering psychosis.

What we are looking for here is to use it for medical purposes e.g., for managing **anxiety** and **chronic pain**. Literally hundreds of different chemicals have been isolated from these versatile plants.[2] Of these, the most common oils used medically are Cannabidiol (CBD) oil and tetrahydrocannabinol (THC) oil. They can be used alone or in combination and it is also worth noting, have anti-inflammatory properties which may assist with reducing the brain inflammation noted in ME/CFS.

CBD oil is readily available as it is not considered psychoactive, and therefore is not considered addictive and can be purchased for personal use. I found it particularly helpful for anxiety.

If pain is the main issue then a combination of THC and CBD may work best. I suggest if you wish to try medicinal cannabis or at least explore this option further, then locate a practitioner experienced with prescribing this; a compounding pharmacist may be able to direct you to one.

Integrative Medicine

What I've described above are examples as they might apply to ME/CFS of the huge area of Integrative or Functional Medicine. Apart from training in conventional medicine, an integrative medicine practitioner is a medical doctor who has extra training in complementary therapies and other functional medicines, sometimes administering them intravenously.

A reminder for those attracted to exploring this further just be aware of your budget, as it can involve expensive testing and ongoing supplement expenses. If you're interested in exploring this approach further, there are Integrative Medicine Associations in the UK, Europe and the USA. In Australia, you might like to look up the Australian Integrative Medicine Association (AIMA) at http://aima.net.au and see if they can direct you to a suitable practitioner.

Most integrative medicine doctors have their own special areas of interest, but generally someone with ME/CFS would receive the following approach:

1. Assessment would include blood and urine testing and then depending on results, if appropriate, optimizing the bodies endocrine (hormone) systems with medication;
2. Treating previously undetected infections, such as candida (a yeast) overgrowth; mold exposure;

3. Reducing inflammation;
4. Enhancing detoxification pathways;
5. and refreshing the microbiome through diet and supplementation. Let me share some further examples.

Diet and Dysbiosis

There is evidence that people affected by ME/CFS have an unhealthy balance of bowel bugs (dysbiosis) when compared with healthy people. The importance of a healthy gut microbiome (population of bugs) in achieving good health is becoming increasingly recognized for a wide range of illnesses.[3-5] Increasing vegetable and fruit intake and fiber generally is the key to improving one's microbiome. From a treatment perspective, in some people with ME/CFS diet can be the critical missing link. In Chapters 8 and 9 we will have a comprehensive look at diet.

DHEA

One potential integrative medicine I have personally experienced is taking the **adrenal** hormone, Dehydroepiandrosterone (DHEA). This is sometimes prescribed if your naturally occurring DHEA-S is found to be low on a blood test. Whilst in the United States, DHEA can be purchased from a health food store, in Australia this hormone is available on prescription only from a compounding pharmacist. While I am unaware of any placebo controlled clinical trials that support the use of DHEA in treating ME/CFS, in his book, *On Hope and Healing*, U.S. MD Neil Nathan, describes the successful use of DHEA over a 20-year period.[6] In this time his clinic has treated over 5000 patients found to have low DHEA-S on blood testing, Supplementation has brought improvements in immune function, stamina and well-being.

His experience is that noticeable benefits occur within weeks or months and if it is beneficial, he recommends an ongoing prescription period of 12 months to 'kickstart' the adrenal glands.

I had my DHEA levels tested and they were low. Subsequently I found supplementing with DHEA improved my energy levels significantly within three weeks. There are some contraindications to its use, so it is best taken under the supervision of an integrative medical practitioner. I'm unaware of any endocrinology (hormone) specialists who recommend this treatment for ME/CFS management. This said, the endocrinologist who helped manage my thyroid condition agreed my DHEA level was low and accepted that I felt better for supplementing with it.

Nutritional Supplements

First off, let me say that the use of supplements should ideally be supervised by a knowledgeable health professional. Because people affected by ME/CFS often eat so poorly, as they can lack the finances to afford healthy food and the energy for shopping and food preparation, they may benefit from a multivitamin/multimineral. Research suggests this can indeed improve symptoms.[7]

Vitamin D3 Levels should be checked as a baseline as people affected by ME/CFS are at risk for osteoporosis due to lack of weight bearing exercise, lack of sunlight exposure and poor gut absorption. Low vitamin D levels can contribute to muscle pain and Fibromyalgia. In some instances, this pain can completely resolve within weeks of introducing a Vitamin D supplement.[8] There is also growing evidence suggesting adequate vitamin D levels protect you against respiratory infections[9] and help in managing serious hospitalized COVID-19 infections.[10]

When you're getting a blood test for a vitamin D level, check vitamin

B12 and folate levels as well.

Supplementing with Vitamin B12 and B-complex can be helpful although you may need to use the activated forms. Let me explain.

Methylation Defects

Both **B12 and folate** play important roles in many hundreds of chemical reactions within our body's cells. In particular, researchers have focused on their role in a biochemical process known as methylation. Methylation plays many important roles including detoxification, DNA repair and energy metabolism. Defective or weak methylating ability can be detected on genetic testing and has been linked with the development of many chronic illnesses.

Patients with ME/CFS have been found to have low levels of B12 and high levels of homocysteine (I'll explain in a moment) in their cerebrospinal fluid (the fluid that bathes the brain and spinal cord).[11] If your B12 is low, a trial of B12, methylcobalamin, 1000 µg via intramuscular injection weekly for 6 weeks may be helpful. Importantly, this needs to be combined with an oral folic acid supplement. Fatigue and cognitive symptoms may improve and if this is going to help, you will know within a few weeks. Cognitive improvement was dramatic for some of my patients whose B12 levels tested low or in the lower levels of what was considered normal. Apart from local soreness/skin reactions at the injection sites, I am unaware of any reported side effects, despite the high B12 blood levels achieved by these injections.[12]

One study involving 38 people affected by ME/CFS, confirmed a long-term benefit (up to 20 years and an average of 8 years in patients who responded well) for ongoing regular injections of B12 combined with oral folic acid tablets, particularly when higher doses were used.[13] A possible explanation for the benefits of this treatment could relate to improvements in methylation.

The Methylation Pathway

The effectiveness of folate utilization in promoting healthy methylation is largely determined by how efficient an enzyme in the body known as Methylenetetrahydrofolate Reductase (MTHFR) is operating.[14,15] Luckily you don't have to pronounce it to make it work!

If MTHFR is sluggish however, then any folate absorbed by the body will be less effective in preventing the build-up in the bloodstream of a chemical known as homocysteine. High levels of homocysteine produce inflammation via oxidative stress, a chemical process (like 'rusting') which is damaging to various body cells, including those of the cardiovascular system and the brain.[16] Dosing up on B vitamins has been shown to increase blood folate levels and lower homocysteine levels if they are high.[17,18]

If you wish to look at your methylation efficiency, it would be best if you worked with an integrative medicine doctor trained in this area who can individualize your testing and treatment. When I had a blood test to determine my MTHFR status, I discovered that I had the C677T homozygous variety (i.e., the most sluggish version that operates at 20-30% of the efficiency of the healthiest version). This version is found in 5 to 15% of the population. To improve my body's methylation performance, I now take an activated B complex which includes MTHFR.

Essential Fatty Acid Supplements

Given we now know that neuroinflammation is present in people with ME/CFS, it makes sense to make sure our diet has enough anti-inflammatory omega 3 fatty acids in it. Fish, chia seeds and walnuts are good sources of omega 3s. Supplementation with Essential Fatty Acids (EFA's) can also improve symptoms for some people affected by ME/CFS. This is particularly so with supplementation with eicosapentanoic acid (EPA) and Docosahexaenoic Acid (DHA), essential fatty acids found in omega-3 fish oil, which has been shown to resolve neuro-inflammation.[19-21]

Other Supplements

Vitamin and mineral cofactors including vitamin C, biotin, niacin, selenium, zinc, and magnesium (which can help reduce muscle cramps especially if taken before bed), may be supportive in conjunction with EFA's. Zinc deficiency may contribute to decreased function of natural killer cells (a finding in people with ME/CFS – see *ME/CFS A Doctor's Journey Ch 12)* and cell-mediated immune dysfunction.[22] Zinc supplements must be balanced with copper in the correct ratio so get personalized advice on this.

Blood levels of **coenzyme Q 10** (CoQ10), which plays an important role in mitochondrial energy production, are significantly lower in a substantial number of people affected by ME/CFS compared to healthy controls. Some patients may show improvement with CoQ10 supplementation of 100–400 mg daily. If effective, to maintain improvement, CoQ10 needs to be taken long term.[23,24] A caution here, this can be expensive.

Preliminary research into supplementation with **D-ribose**, a carbohydrate naturally found within the body, which is also used in mitochondrial energy production, has been promising. In a study conducted by Dr Jacob Teitelbaum and colleagues, a dosage of 5 g of D-ribose powder three times a day was given to 257 people with ME/CFS and/or Fibromyalgia. After just 3 weeks, there was a 61.7% reported average improvement in energy levels, with a 37% average improvement in well-being. Significant improvements in sleep (29.3 %), mental clarity (30%) and pain intensity (16.6%) were also reported.[24]

CHAPTER 4 INTEGRATING COMPLEMENTARY THERAPIES (CT'S)

It should be noted, whilst promising, this was not a placebo-controlled trial. If you are attracted to having your own trial of D-ribose, you should use the n-of-1 approach and will know after three weeks whether or not it is going to help you. If it does, then you can reduce the dose from 5 g three times a day to 5 g twice a day (i.e., after the initial 3 weeks).

Dr Jacob Teitelbaum whose research into D-ribose I'm citing above, is an integrative US physician who suffered and overcame ME/CFS and has published research and books on how his clinic approaches the treatment of people with Fibromyalgia and ME/CFS.[25-27] Reading his book, *The Fatigue and Fibromyalgia Solution*, I was impressed to learn that while he has his own range of nutritional supplements, he claims not to receive any money from the products he recommends, instead donating all profits made from the sale of products he makes available to his patients, to charity.

My own view on practitioners prescribing and selling products from their clinic is that it can be difficult to remain objective in your advice. So, with some exceptions, beware practitioners selling you bucket loads of products!

Your Own N-of-1 Trial

If you are guided to take a complementary therapy (CT), I suggest you rate weekly your symptoms in your Appendix 2 questionnaire before and then after commencing one CT at a time, for one or two months. Note any changes or no changes. Then stop the CT for the same time period noting any symptom change again. Then once again re-institute the same CT treatment seeing if it makes a difference. This should give you a better idea if its worth persisting with for a longer course of time.

This may be the best evidence you can find as clinical research into CT's and ME/CFS is inadequate and so it's possible you'll be paying for expensive placebos. Not that I have a problem with this necessarily, the placebo-effect can be powerful, averaging a 30% benefit.[28] Just be smart and trial the less expensive CTs first!

Katie's story, presented in Chapter 14, in which she was spending hundreds of dollars weekly on expensive natural therapies and not improving prior to attending the Austin Hospital ME/CFS program, is a cautionary tale about believing natural therapies alone will provide a miracle cure.

Chapter 4
Key Points

- ✓ My experience is that CT's can improve symptoms and support a Rehab approach, but alone are not as effective as Rehab in bringing about lasting change.
- ✓ There are promising areas of CT research, but more research is required.
- ✓ If you wish to explore these approaches further the Australian Integrative Medicine Association could direct you to an integrative medicine practitioner with a special interest in ME/CFS.
- ✓ Be aware of the expense involved and what your budget is as the cost of testing and the ongoing use of supplements can mount up.

Chapter 5
CHOICE & PROGRESS

"The first step is often the hardest...."
ANONYMOUS

Where to Begin?

In Appendix 2, I have included a questionnaire which I suggest you fill in. This lists the most common problems people with ME/CFS tend to experience. Rank their severity from 1 to 20 by placing a number in the [ ] on the left hand side of the symptom and then rate the severity of each from 0 to 3. This can help you, your carer and your assisting health practitioner to prioritize which areas to target first.

Keep a journal repeating this questionnaire every 3 months, on the first Sunday of each new season, noting any differences. If things are improving, focus on how far you've come. If things are not improving or going the wrong way, then you need to share this with your GP who might need to reassess the diagnosis or suggest a different approach.

The holistic terrain-improving program itself is flexible; you can begin to address ME/CFS from different directions. While this book can be worked through from cover to cover, its best to individualize your direction. This will be guided by the problems identified in your answers to the questionnaire, what your health practitioner identifies and your current life circumstances. It will also be influenced by what you have tried and read up until now.

I have structured the chapters to ensure your understanding of ME/CFS continues to grow throughout your reading of this book. If you are still unsure of where to begin, my experience is that it is best you start with the fundamental four: Social Support; Restorative Sleep; Nourishing Diet; and Movement.

Social Support

It may require you to reach out to others and take some time by building an understanding social network of **support**, ideally family and/or friends and health care providers, is your best chance at improving your situation. If they are capable of understanding what's going on as well as being helpful on practical and/or emotional levels, then we know this can increase your chances of restoring your quality of life and underpin the other aspects of terrain building. If not, you'll need to look elsewhere and an ME/CFS support group in person or online is a good place to start.

Restorative Sleep

As it is becoming increasingly apparent a lack of refreshing **sleep** can be a primary or secondary player in most people with ME/CFS, so it is worthwhile addressing issues with sleep early on. Up to 50% of people with ME/CFS have or go on to develop sleep apnea.

Maximizing Nutririon

Adequate **nutrition** is essential for supporting your terrain. It can also improve symptoms along with increasing the variety of good bacteria in your gut, the microbiome. In my own case, energy swings that had related to sweet foods and refined carbohydrates improved markedly when I shifted to a low GI diet. In Alexandra Barton's book[1] there were four people (out of 50) who attributed their recovery largely due to the 'no whites' low GI diet.

Movement

When it comes to **movement**, the final member of the foundation four, I suggest you look at **pacing,** Micro-Rehab and the Rest/Activity dance. Pacing of activities with strategic rest periods is an important strategy for managing fatigue and pain. It is much underrated and a lifelong skill that can allow your body to strengthen and prevent or at least minimize setbacks.

Loops of Fear

If you are very anxious about introducing more physical movement into your life, often due to previous bad experiences with Post-exertional Malaise (PEM), then I suggest you look at Chapter 13 where you can learn the art of mindful relaxation, the 'rest' aspect of the Rest/Activity dance. Then I'd suggest you read Chapter 15 Defuse the Loop. Here you will learn not only how to rest, but how to settle fears and mental agitation. There is an inner battle we need to overcome as part of ME/CFS management, but don't stress, there are some simple ways we can do this.

People with ME/CFS, myself included, often do not realize that fearful thoughts are occurring in the background. Whether they be triggered by neuroinflammation or simply due to a secondary effect of freaking out about an illness that appears to have us trapped, we don't know. Whatever the cause, this creates loops of fear that release fight/flight chemicals that unbalance our terrain, locking us in, as recurring fight/flight loops keep us from any chance of improving. Fortunately, and surprisingly perhaps, once identified these can be readily defused, allowing your pacing and Micro-Rehab to be far more effective.

Growing your Intuition

The application of the information you will learn in Chapters 13-15 will be like compost to your garden, growing your intuition so that it becomes more accessible to you. In the future your ability to choose what's best for you will become clearer and easier.

Mapping Your Progress - Get Creative!

Monitoring your own progress can be helpful, especially if you're about to introduce a new treatment approach. In this way you can see if anything is changing. This is the backbone to your n-of-1 'suck it and see' research. I am aware of Apps being developed to monitor symptoms but the only one available as I type is one specifically for pacing, an area we will look at in Chapter 10.

It may help you to share this Progress Map with your health practitioners or carers who can also provide feedback on your progress.

Depending on the treatment being trialed, some people like to jot this down daily or weekly. Others prefer a longer-term view only, recording monthly or even three monthly (e.g., after changing your diet). You can of course combine this by, for example, having weekly monitoring for a short time after a course of say, vitamin B12, and then monthly after this.

It is up to you to decide what makes you feel the best. Some people find monitoring themselves too often can make them more anxious. If this occurs, no biggie, just lengthen the view or stop. Some people will switch off at this point as making charts and monitoring themselves is not their thing. That's completely up to you but I'd suggest getting creative if that helps you to engage with this. Remember this is to help **you** to see how you are travelling, so that in time you'll see how far you've come. If it's worrying you out though, or not helping, either stop, (yes, I mean it – it's not essential) or try another way.

CHAPTER 5 CHOICE & PROGRESS

In the example given below, Caitlin (her story appears in Chapter 6) was rating each symptom numerically between 1 and 3 on a weekly basis (around sunset each Sunday for 4 weeks). A score of zero meant absent and 3 meant severe. Notice the effects on her brain fog (poor concentration) of restoring her low Vitamin B12 levels. See Table 1 below.

Symptoms	**Sun Oct 6**	**Sun Oct 13**	**Sun Oct 20**	**Sun Oct 27**	**Comments**
Fatigue	3	3	2	3	
Pain	2	2	2	3	
Unrefreshing - Sleep	3	3	2	3	
Brain Fog	3	1	1	1	Since 3rd B 12 injection Wed Oct 9 Improved
Dizziness when upright	3	3	2	3	
Anxiety	3	2	2	2	

Table 1 Caitlin's weekly Symptom (After Vit B 12) Check 0 = absent 3 = severe

Others, like myself, preferred a tick chart to mark where one simply marks off positive activities at the end or during each day. That way, even on 'tough' days, you can see that you are still doing something towards helping yourself to restore more life. See Table 2 below. I did this for the initial three months of my rehab program to help me to keep on track.

Of course, there is nothing stopping you having both a daily chart to mark and say a monthly or three-monthly symptom checking chart as well.

So, before you start to introduce the terrain building plan, see if you can draw up a spread sheet relevant to your situation. For the more mathematically minded you may wish to graph your progress every 1 to 3 months (see Fig 1. Squiggly CFS Progress graph).

Activity	Oct 8th	Oct 9th	Oct 10th	Oct 11th	Oct 12th	Oct 13th	Oct 14th	Oct 15th	Comments
Deep breathing	****	******	***	*****	***	****	******	*****	Before meals and bedtime
Positive Emotional Thoughts (PETS) approx	10 x	4 x	30 x	30 x	10 x	5 x	20 x	10 x	(see Ch?)
Walk to post box	2x	3 x	3 x	x	2 x	2 x	-	2 x	Pedometer avg 750
Meditation	5 min	10 min	5min x2	5 min x2	10 min	-	5 min x2	5 min	Sleep better

TABLE 2 My daily chart (for positive inputs)

What to Expect

The restoring process with ME/CFS is rarely a straight line. To begin with, it is usually more like a rollercoaster with ups and downs, indicating setbacks from time to time (see Figure 1 ME/CFS Progress squiggly graph). At Point A you might feel terrible, point B much better and overdo it, causing you to crash down to Point C where you feel like you are back at the beginning again. Then as you apply your new skills you restore faster and have more good days, then you'll head to Point D, a much healthier and more enjoyable place to be, with only occasional smaller setbacks.

The key here is to remember that setbacks are part of the process and not to become disheartened. If you are keeping a journal of your progress you can comment on what you believe was the cause of the setback and learn from it. In time, the depth of setbacks will become less and less as you become more skilled in managing your energy envelope and pacing. This will allow you to restore more smoothly than would otherwise have been possible and build both physical and emotional stamina again.

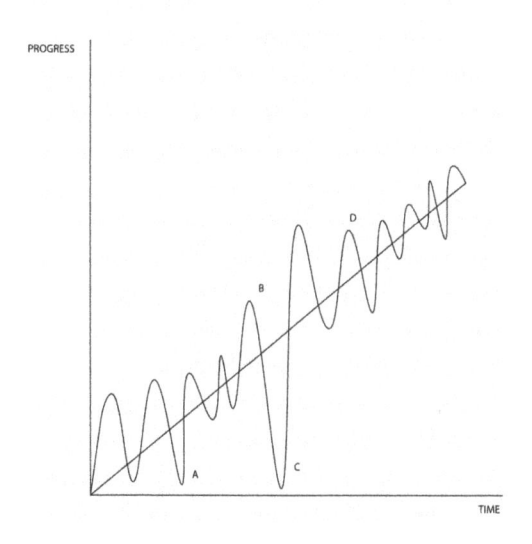

Figure 1. Squiggly Line of Progress Graph.

The Daily Scorecard/Emoji

Some people with ME/CFS, who live with their carer's, partner and/or others, found giving them a scorecard indicative of how they were feeling at the beginning of each day (i.e., from 1 to 10 or some prefer Emoji's) would help direct their behaviour.

So, for example, if you were feeling unwell a score of 3 (grumpy/sad face Emoji) would give the household the message not to be as chatty and keep things quieter and more restful that day. The scorecard would also allow you not to have to explain your need for time out all the time. If others lived in the household at different hours of the day, this scorecard could be placed in a position, say on the fridge or written on a whiteboard, where everyone could see it. In this situation, the carer, rather than the person with ME/CFS needing to rest, could take on the role of letting others know, returning phone calls/texts etc.

Chapter 5
Key Points

- ✓ This book is written in such a way that it can be read from cover to cover. There is flexibility, however, depending upon what you have learnt in the past, as you can upend ME/CFS from different starting points.
- ✓ Once you have read to this point you can then decide which order to look at the remaining chapters.
- ✓ Regardless of where you begin, you will need to learn the art of Pacing.
- ✓ There are different ways of monitoring and mapping your progress. I have shared a few in this chapter, including symptom questionnaires and journaling three monthly to a daily tick chart of positive activities. Choose a way that encourages you. If it is making you more anxious, or pressured then either try a different way, discuss with friends or health practitioners' other ways that might suit you better, or just stop the monitoring but continue on with the program.
- ✓ To relieve stress during bad days consider using a daily scorecard or emoji to alert others. Stick it on your fridge.

Chapter 6

REACHING OUT - BUILDING SOCIAL SCAFFOLDING

> *"From what I've seen, it isn't so much the act of asking that paralyses us--it's what lies beneath: the fear of being vulnerable, the fear of rejection, the fear of looking needy or weak. The fear of being seen as a burdensome member of the community instead of a productive one."*
>
> **AMANDA PALMER, THE ART OF ASKING; OR, HOW I LEARNED TO STOP WORRYING AND LET PEOPLE HELP[1]**

Caitlin's Story

Caitlin was 43 years old and married with two young sons when I first consulted with her in 2008. Three years prior to this she was diagnosed with ME/CFS and Fibromyalgia. These conditions had developed on a background of working in a high-pressure administrative officer's position, postnatal depression and a nasty attack of viral meningitis that had required hospitalization. Following this triggering meningitis attack, she suffered persistent and severe headaches and generalized muscle pain and fatigue. Other symptoms included post-exertional malaise, anxiety, unrefreshing sleep, brain fog with impaired concentration, irritable bowel syndrome and an irritable bladder, dizziness and the loss of adaptability and tolerance for stress. All symptoms worsened in the second half of her menstrual cycle, culminating in dreadful period pain.

Post-exertional malaise and fatigue were particularly difficult problems for Caitlin. Any excessive physical or emotional exertion would commonly leave her unwell for the next four or five days or longer. For example, a visit from her sister from interstate would be both enjoyable and exhausting. Caitlin also struggled to keep up with her two growing sons, becoming overwhelmed by their needs and leaving her, at times, bedridden with pain. This extreme pain and limitation could take the form of migraine, back pain, chronic neck pain, with difficulties lifting, bending and sometimes even showering.

Her situation was seriously compounded by the fact that her husband and extended family did not believe in the severity of her illness and the limitations it imposed upon her. Her attempts to explain the situation were met with sideways looks, changing the subject or an uninformed remark such as, 'get your act together, I get tired too.' She expressed feeling 'damaged' by their incongruent responses to her situation and even wished she'd had cancer because that would have brought more empathy.

Caitlin had tried numerous things to get well before consulting with me, including 12 months of weekly counselling sessions with a therapist trained in 'Reverse therapy.' If anything, her condition had only worsened. Despite these backward steps, throughout the three years in which I consulted with Caitlin, I found her to be highly motivated and an active participant in her own management. I introduced her to pacing, stress management, mind-body cognitive strategies and I referred her to an exercise physiologist with experience in treating people with ME/CFS.

I invited Caitlin to bring her husband along to a consultation. She sat beside him whilst I explained the reality of ME/CFS and the challenges it posed for her. Following this, he developed a greater understanding and compassion for her suffering. During this time, Caitlin also attended a chiropractor and a psychiatrist who placed her on an antidepressant medication (a selective serotonin re-uptake inhibitor (SSRI)). Caitlin also undertook a series of Botox injections into muscles around her head and neck to reduce migraine, jaw and neck pain. This gave her some temporary relief. In a further attempt to improve her situation, she even underwent a hysterectomy. This cured her of her painful menstruation but did not impact upon her ME/CFS or Fibromyalgia symptoms.

She had times of improvement, sometimes lasting for several months, but would then relapse in response to a physical or emotional stress. Nine years after her original diagnosis, she has been unable to return to work and her husband has lost his job. Bravely, they decided to sell their home and move their young family interstate to be closer to a more supportive sibling and further away from destructive, disbelieving inputs from Caitlin's mother and other siblings. At our last interaction (by phone) she was particularly relieved to be distancing herself from her mother and was looking forward to a brighter life in Queensland.

Going where the openings are

Caitlin's story demonstrates how a supportive framework could either make or break us. Her setbacks were often related to disrespectful interactions with family. In the end she saw she'd have no chance of recovery in this environment and had to get away. The social context is often overlooked as the most powerful influencer of our body's terrain. Yet, as you may recall from *A Doctor's Journey Back to Health Ch 9*, in 1988 the prestigious journal, Science, concluded that having a lack of emotional support in your life was a greater risk factor for disease and death than smoking.[2] This came on the back of research that demonstrated the most lonely and isolated had three to four times the risk of dying prematurely when compared with those with close social ties.[3,4]

Whilst we all have different personalities and needs in terms of social interactions, this illness tends to turn relationships on their head asking of us to negotiate a 'new normal.' For instance, if you are a person who others once relied upon for support you will now need to accept your limitations and allow others to support you. This can be tricky for you and them, so, do not be surprised if they cannot. Yet, if you are going to have any chance of improving it is critical you put yourself first now and if possible, choose to interact/hang out with people who believe in you and your ability to improve. Be gentle with yourself, though, it will take time for you to learn your body's capacities and then to be honest both in expressing your need for connection as well as expressing how much time/energy you have for these interactions. Initially you may only manage a few minutes on the phone.

In my own case, choosing to interact with people who accepted the 'new' broken me was difficult. Letting them know that my ability to interact would be limited was very hard for me and later, most of my ME/CFS patients, to learn and express. Not everyone is going to be able to respond to you and you may need let go of previously 'close friends' if they continue to demand your energy and attention. This is tough.

In the end though you are going to need to go where the openings are, as Caitlin did, where you feel nurtured and able to cope. If the old social scaffolding is unable to adequately support you, you will need to be proactive and seek out new supports.

Support groups

A few words about support groups. Given the many misconceptions about ME/CFS, it's no surprise that a key role that ME/CFS support groups play is to validate the reality of the illness. Some also play an invaluable role in directing people towards local doctors and other practitioners with an understanding of the condition. In addition, they can provide educational materials that can help to explain what

CHAPTER 6   REACHING OUT - BUILDING SOCIAL SCAFFOLDING

is going on to family and friends. Some groups also provide education about management, such as pacing.

Whether or not you are inclined to attend such a group, or participate online, depends very much on your circumstance and personality. An advantage of online communities is that you can choose to step away more easily once you've expressed yourself and acknowledged others. When I attended a local ME/CFS support group, I witnessed that some members of the group felt at home there and had made friendships that sustained them. My own experience was different. I could see the overwhelming need of each person, including myself, to have the reality of their horrendous situation affirmed. This was clearly critical, but I also found the experience to be exhausting and decided not to re-attend for this reason.

This contrasted with my experience of attending another support group for Parkinson's disease (PD), an illness I developed much later. Parkinson's Disease needs no extra validation as it is already recognized as a chronic debilitating disease and is 'valid' in the eyes of society and the medical profession. Here, even though the illness was difficult to bear and disabling, the focus in these groups was more relaxed and fun. We didn't have to waste energy on restoring validity; that was a given. The fact that PD had a range of established pharmaceuticals and/or surgical treatment options created an easy point of focus too. ME/CFS had none of this.

These fundamental differences go some way to explaining the research finding that ME/CFS patients often do worse if they attend an ME/CFS support group.[5,6] I believe it's likely that the group attracts those people with the least amount of social support who would have been even worse off without a support group. I certainly found this in my clinic. In fact, I only recommended a support group for those desperately in need of it. Those who had good supports, after having their illness validated by their doctor (i.e., me), were able to take the next step and focus their limited energy on ways to best improve their health.

To finish this discussion about support groups, let me just say that each individual group will have a different dynamic, so the only way to fully know if it will be helpful for you or not, is to do what I did and check it out. Like me, you may decide to only attend once, or you might become an occasional or regular attendee, you be the judge of what works best for you.

Support Groups Push Ahead Research

Because of the long history of ME/CFS being derided as a malingering illness there is a great deal of emphasis in many support groups to focus on research demonstrating its reality. This has been very positive in helping to drive biomedical research into the condition and has now led to its greater recognition as a real biomedical illness.

A cautionary note here though. Many ME/CFS groups have been battling for recognition for decades and it will take more years for them to gain trust that society will become a safe place for them as the growing body of evidence, the awareness of long Covid and its connection to ME/CFS, or indeed the 2015 pronouncement by the Institute of Medicine (National Academy of Medicine – as it is now known -See *A Doctor's Journey Back to Health Ch 12*) that ME/CFS is a biomedical disease takes hold in mainstream medicine.

Until the biomedical reality of the illness is common knowledge to the medical profession, their friends, family and acquaintances and in every loungeroom across the world they will continue to fight for recognition and rightly so.

This has led some ME/CFS groups to dismiss all evidence that people can and do improve their health despite a diagnosis with the illness. Perhaps in their minds, if people can improve, it undermines the continued attempts to validate the illness as a biomedical one rather

CHAPTER 6 REACHING OUT - BUILDING SOCIAL SCAFFOLDING

than the old unfounded perception of it as a hysterical disorder (see *A Doctor's Journey Back to Health, Chapter 2 - A Brief History of ME/CFS.*). Therefore, if you attend these groups and your condition improves, or you aim to recover some or much of the life you'd lost it may be difficult for your diagnosis of ME/CFS to seem credible to them, even though most other neurological diseases do improve with appropriate terrain strategies.

So, do not let this derail your efforts to improve your condition using the strategies outlined in this book. As I've said before, one day there may be a scientifically validated specific medical treatment or medication for ME/CFS but in the meantime there are lots of evidenced based 'terrain' measures that can be implemented and will synergize together to improve your situation. Remember many of these same measures are already considered medical best practice in the restoration of function for people with other 'validated' chronic illnesses.

The reality is that some people's situation is such that it's very difficult to even attempt this 'terrain improving' approach. Remember there is a spectrum of severity and the longer you have the illness the more difficult it is to maintain or obtain the sustained social support you'd need to have a chance of major improvement. That said, don't let this put you off, people like Caitlin who have been severely unwell for years are some of the strongest most motivated people I've ever met and was proactive in seeking social support and achieved the reward.

So, let's turn to the other terrain strategies that will help you find your path back to life.

Chapter 6
Key Points

- ✓ The social context we find ourselves in is one of the most powerful influences on our terrain.
- ✓ Being proactive in seeking help takes courage but is critical if you are to build the social support scaffolding for a better life.
- ✓ ME/CFS Support groups either online or in person can be helpful, but not always so. The only way to know is to reach out and see if or which group may work for you.

Chapter 7

RESTORATIVE SLEEP – RECLAIMING NIGH NIGH'S

> *"Even a soul submerged in sleep is hard at work and helps make something of the world."*
> **HERACLITUS,** FRAGMENTS

A good night's sleep can be delicious and refreshing. Yet sadly this is not easily obtained with this illness. Unrefreshing sleep is one of the hallmarks of ME/CFS. Research confirms that people with ME/CFS take longer to fall asleep, spend a longer time in bed and have less deep refreshing sleep than healthy people.[1] They also have higher levels of anxiety which in both people with ME/CFS and healthy people is associated with worse sleep quality.[2]

If one is to improve this, it helps to understand sleep better.

The Autonomic Nervous System

The quality of our sleep is linked to the healthy function of the Autonomic Nervous System (ANS). The ANS operates all the time without us being aware of it keeping our hearts beating and our bodies breathing while we are awake or asleep. It does so from its home base in the brainstem, orchestrating impulses from the sympathetic (fight/flight) and parasympathetic (rest/digest) nervous systems. These impulses travel via nerve fibres down the spinal cord and beyond to all our vital organs.

One measure of the health of the ANS is heart rate variability (HRV). It may sound counter-intuitive, but it is healthier to have a slightly irregular heartbeat than one more like a metronome. Increased HRV means more variability and indicates greater parasympathetic nervous system activity. This is a good thing as its associated with better sleep, improved mood, a stronger more balanced immune system and greater resilience to stress.

Research also reports that in people with ME/CFS, overnight parasympathetic activity is decreased relative to sympathetic activity, indicating the body and mind are working harder than they should. This reduces Heart Rate Variability and is the inverse of what should be occurring during rest. This pattern has been linked to unrefreshing sleep in ME/CFS and other conditions.[3-5] Fortunately, one can change this.

The Sleep Cycle

There is a wide variation in terms of the hours of sleep we each need per night. Whilst we tend to need less sleep as we age, on average, in order to feel refreshed, a healthy adult needs eight hours of quality sleep; adolescents, nine hours. Over this period we cycle through five stages of sleep around four times. The deeper dreamless non-REM (rapid eye movement) sleep occurs earlier on in the night, whilst the lighter dream-filled REM sleep increases progressively with each cycle as the world outside moves closer to dawn (Figure 1).

While no one is sure of the mechanism of how ME/CFS causes poorer quality sleep, preliminary evidence suggests that abnormal alterations in sleep stage transitions may contribute.

CHAPTER 7 RESTORATIVE SLEEP – RECLAIMING NIGH NIGH'S

Sleep Cycles

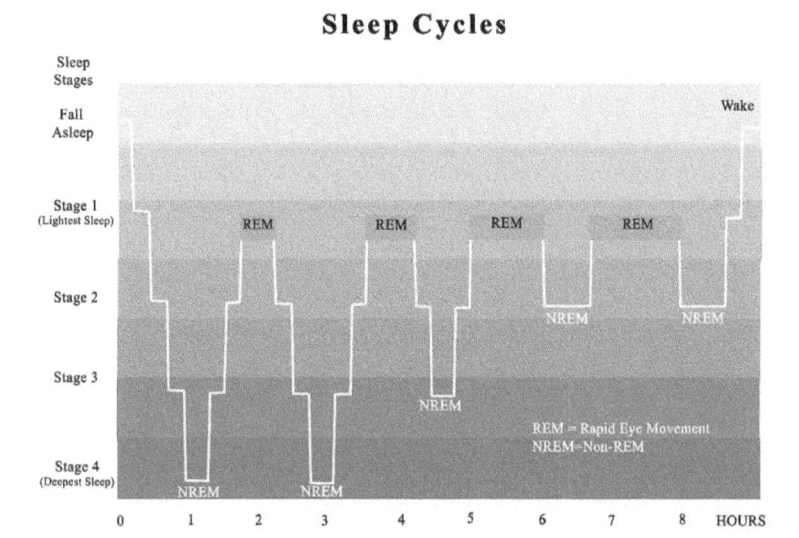

Figure 1. A Healthy Sleep Pattern Hypnogram. Notice how the length of time (on the horizontal x axis) spent in REM sleep increases as sleep cycles progress over a night, while the deepest (Stage 4) sleep stages occur early-on, within the first 1 to 3 hours after falling to sleep.

During rapid eye movement (REM) sleep there is, as the name suggests, darting movements of the eyes under closed eyelids. Brain waves during REM sleep appear very similar to brain waves during wakefulness (See Figure 2 and Table 1). In contrast, non-REM (NREM) sleep is subdivided into four stages distinguished from each other and from wakefulness by characteristic patterns of brain waves. The first four stages of sleep are NREM sleep, while the fifth and final stage of sleep is REM sleep.

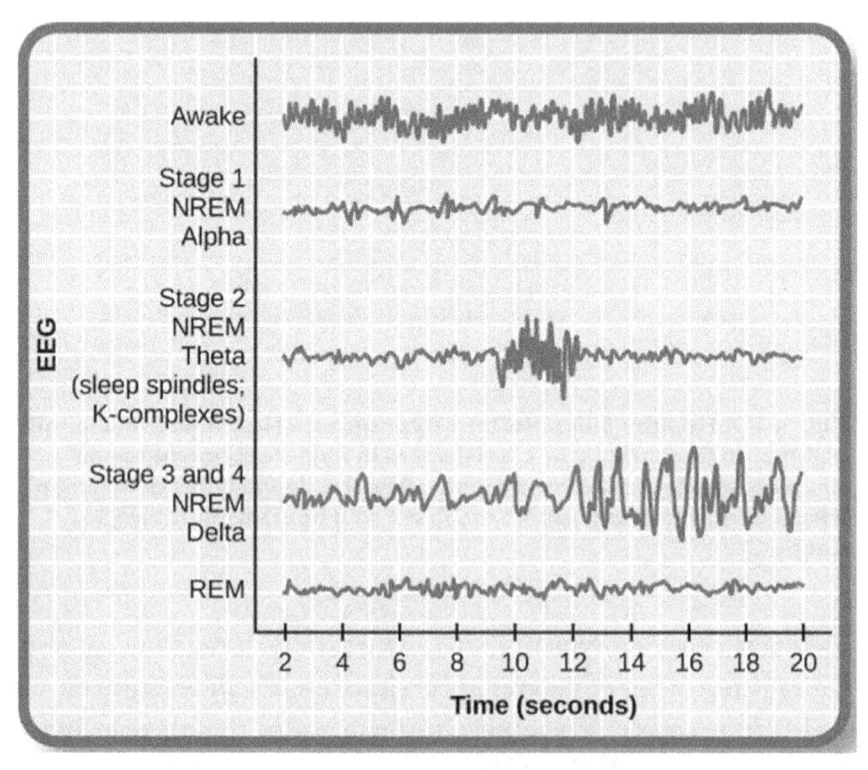

Figure 2. Electro-encephalograms (EEG) demonstrates how brainwave activity changes dramatically across the five different stages of sleep.

Gamma Brainwaves:	
	- Frequency: 32 – 100 Hz (Fastest) - State of mind: Heightened perception, learning, problem-solving tasks
Beta Brainwaves:	
	- Frequency: 13-32 Hz - State of mind: Alert, normal alert consciousness, active thinking
Alpha Brainwaves:	
	- Frequency: 8-13 Hz - State of mind: Physically and mentally relaxed
Theta Brainwaves:	
	- Frequency: 4-8 Hz - State of mind: Creativity, insight, meditation, daydreams, reduced consciousness
Delta Brainwaves:	
	- Frequency: 0.5-4 Hz (Slowest) - State: Sleep, non-dreaming, restorative

Table 1 Five Brainwaves

The occurrence of REM too soon after sleep onset, referred to as Sleep Onset REM Period or SOREMP, is considered abnormal and is one cause of unrefreshing sleep in ME/CFS.[3]

Another common finding in people with ME/CFS is a flattening of the normal peaks and troughs seen on a healthy overnight hypnogram (See Figure 1).

How much REM Sleep do you need?

Too little REM sleep can leave you feeling groggy, less focussed, and with memory problems. That's why it's important to get enough sleep after learning something new or before taking an exam. Some medications can also block REM sleep by half (such as some antidepressants).

Too much REM can also create problems, like too much brain activation, leaving you angry, irritable, and may contribute to the symptoms of depression and anxiety.

What about Deep Stage 4 Sleep?

There's no real way to get too much deep sleep. The body has its own natural drive for deep sleep, and once it gets enough and the need for it decreases, the body just goes into REM and light sleep.[4]

Sleep disorders can keep you out of deep sleep and make sleep a little shallower. Your body wants to get into deep sleep at night, and it wants to avoid deep sleep during the day. There is a natural delay of how long it will take you to get into it.

Electro-encephalograms, EEG's, have also detected **sleep instability** in people with ME/CFS where a brain wave that is normally present in awake people who have their eyes closed, disrupts the deeper phases of sleep causing restlessness and potentially waking people up, like an internal alarm clock set too early. This is called **alpha-wave intrusion**.[5]

Other physiological mechanisms, such as abnormal heart rate variability (HRV) and altered cortisol profiles, may also contribute to poorer sleep in ME/CFS. Additionally, poor sleep quality in ME/CFS has been found to be associated with higher levels of the pro-inflammatory cytokines thought to be a cause of most symptoms of ME/CFS[6] (see *A Doctor's Journey back to Health* Chapter 12).

What to Do?

Importantly, it is possible to improve sleep patterns and sleep quality, and this can make a real and beneficial impact on all ME/CFS symptoms. While many scientists are unsure as to why we need to sleep at all, there is little doubt that it has a profound effect on our health and well-being. As sleep expert Dr Merrill Mitler summarizes, "sleep services all aspects of our body in one way or another: molecular, energy balance, as well as intellectual function, alertness and mood."7

Identify Obvious Sleep Disruptors

There are a long list of symptoms that can disrupt your sleep during the night. These include pain, a blocked nose, itchy skin, cramp, overheating, indigestion, an irritable bladder or bowel, restless legs or a general restlessness from feeling ill. There are many ways to address these problems. For example, GP's may prescribe antihistamines or medicated creams for itchy skin. There are also specific medications available for Restless Legs Syndrome.

Saline nasal spray works well for unblocking your nose and helps flush away toxins and viruses. This may have a potential bonus benefit. We know the common cold virus and the COVID-19 virus gain entry via the nose; keeping it flushed with saline may help in prevention (just as washing hands does) and treatment. It is also safe to use regularly.

If the spray is inadequate ask your pharmacist about sinus flow products that douche the back of the nose with liquid saline. Saline can be made at home with the following formula: to 1/3 cup boiling water dissolve a ¼ tsp salt (and ¼ tsp bicarbonate of soda if using in the nose) then add 2/3rd cup cold water.

Dietitians or natural therapists may suggest healthy dietary modifications i.e., too much sugar, wheat and dairy can cause sinus mucus build-up in some people. If you have a cat that sleeps on your bed, cat dander allergy may be an issue. Work with your health practitioner/s or pharmacist to find solutions that work for you.

Some drugs, foods and supplements can cause disrupted sleep and may need to be modified. Vitamin B, for example, can make you more alert and is better to take earlier in the day. Coffee, nicotine, alcohol, illicit stimulants and 'energy' drinks can also be problematic. So, when you see your GP, make sure you bring in all medications and supplements you are taking. Be as honest as you can be. There is no shame in self-medicating to try to improve your situation, but some ways are better than others.

Identify any Sleep Disorders

The field of sleep disorders medicine has become increasingly complex with more than 90 disorders of sleep described, each with clear diagnostic criteria.[8] They can generally be divided into 3 large groups:

1. those producing **insomnia** (complaints of difficulty falling asleep, staying asleep, or non-restorative sleep)
2. those with a primary complaint of **daytime sleepiness**
3. those associated with **disruptive movements/behaviours during sleep** e.g., restless legs, sleep walking (i.e., disorders of arousal.)

Transient insomnia (defined as less than two weeks) is extremely common, afflicting up to 80% of the population. Chronic insomnia affects 15% of the population. People with ME/CFS tend to have chronic insomnia.

If your sleep problems are ongoing despite instituting my Top Seven Tips (see Table 2) below, you may need to explore other medication options or referral to a sleep specialist centre with your doctor. Be aware, however, that some medications, like certain benzodiazepines (e.g., Temazepam) whilst initially effective can mask the real reasons for the insomnia. If used regularly these medications are highly addictive. Withdrawal can cause an unpleasant REM-rebound, SOREMP. Relying on alcohol as a sedative can also have a similar REM-rebound effect when ceased. Not a good idea.

CHAPTER 7 RESTORATIVE SLEEP – RECLAIMING NIGH NIGH'S

Sleep disorders, such as sleep apnea and restless legs syndrome, can mimic ME/CFS or in some cases occur concurrently. A recent research study found more than 50 percent of those people with ME/CFS, whose symptom picture included excessive daytime sleeping, had a sleep disorder.[9] This was diagnosed by polysomnography (PSG), an overnight sleep lab test.

If excessive daytime sleep is a feature of your ME/CFS then it is possible that the diagnosis is actually a sleep disorder or a combination of each. Hence, the researchers concluded that people with ME/CFS with this symptom picture, "should undergo polysomnography, fill in questionnaires and be offered treatment for sleep disorders before the diagnosis of ME/CFS is set."10

Generally speaking, sleep disorders are much easier to treat than ME/CFS. So, if the simple techniques and medications I'll share here, are unhelpful in restoring the quality of your sleep, you may wish to discuss a referral to a sleep specialist with your GP, especially so if excessive daytime sleep is part of your symptom picture.

Note: Both depression and obstructive sleep apnoea can cause early morning waking and daytime sleepiness. If this is your experience be sure to let your GP know.

Biofeedback -Your Own Sleep Lab

There are devices you can purchase, such as rings (e.g., the OURA Ring) you can wear on your finger overnight while they detect and keep a record of your sleep patterns. This record can then be uploaded to an APP on your mobile. In this way you can see for yourself which factors improve your sleep-patterns and which do not. Your own personal sleep 'laboratory,' if you like.[11]

This ring also detects heart rate variability (HRV) and you can see which strategies increase this variability in real time. Increased HRV indicates greater parasympathetic nervous system activation which is associated with improved mood, a stronger more balanced immune system and greater resilience to stress.

This ring could also be helpful in teaching you how to relax during the day. This may only take one to three months, while you come to learn the 'Rest' part of the Rest/Activity dance (See Chapter 13).

A Winning Routine

For most of the people with ME/CFS that I saw, re-establishing a good sleep pattern was a critical piece of the jigsaw for turning their situation around. To do this they needed to establish a winning bedtime routine. Tips for achieving this are shared below and developing a plan that works for you can be very beneficial. Experiment with those that appeal to you and those you think may be most relevant to your situation. (See Table 2)

Do not overwhelm yourself with trying to change all these things in one go. Start with my Top Seven Tips and add one more strategy each week if required.

Medication

For those who need more assistance, I found the medication, amitriptyline, and the natural sleep inducer, melatonin, were useful for some people with ME/CFS.

Melatonin is a hormone produced by the pineal gland, located at the base of the brain. It's concentration in our bloodstream increases in response to a lack of sunlight, preparing us for sleep. It's been found therefore, to be useful for preventing jetlag and for those with Delayed Sleep-wake disorder (DSWD). That's a fancy name for those who, for whatever reason, are night-owls and find it hard to get to sleep.

I found it to be very helpful for people with ME/CFS with this pattern of having trouble falling off to sleep. The smallest dose in tablet or capsule form is usually 2 or 5mg. I suggest you get a compounding pharmacist to make up a liquid dose so you can start at an even smaller dose. When I trialled it for myself, I found I needed just 1 mg to send me off to 'nigh nighs', whilst some of my patients with ME/CFS needed just 0.5 mg.

(see https://www.sleepfoundation.org/articles/melatonin-and-sleep)

Amitriptyline is a tricyclic antidepressant that has been used safely for decades in a small (10mg) night-time dose to assist in reducing muscle pain in fibromyalgia. In this dose it also suppresses REM sleep.[13] This could be helpful for those having an excess of dreamy superficial sleep or early onset REM (SOREMP), preventing them from dropping to the deeper sleep of Stages 3 and 4.

(see https://www.healthline.com/health/sleep/amitriptyline-for-sleep)

There are also other medications and natural therapies that can be tried in the short-term.[14] Discuss these with your health care provider. As mentioned earlier, people affected by ME/CFS are generally very sensitive to medication and herbal treatments. Hence, it is advisable to start at a quarter of the usual dose and build slowly.[15]

If you work on the Wining Tips (See Table 2) at the same time, the supplements or medication will only be needed short-term to help you to reset your sleep cycle and return to medication-free restorative sleep again.

Winning Tips for Better Sleep

My Top Seven

- Wake and get out of bed at the same time every day even if you feel as if you haven't slept. Open the blinds and look at the daylight to retrain the circadian rhythm (Note: Circadian Rhythms are normal human biological and behavioral functions which vary during each 24-hour period. They include the sleep cycle). It may take some weeks to adjust to, but it is worth it in the end, so stick at it.
- Establish a night-time routine so you go to sleep when your body is winding down. Going to bed for example at 10:00 p.m. and waking 7–10 hrs later (depending on the body's needs). This helps maintain healthy circadian rhythms. At night the circadian sleep train arrives approximately every 45 minutes, be ready to 'climb' aboard.
- Avoid electronics i.e., watching TV or using mobiles, computer and other devices with screens for an hour or more before bed. These images are stimulating and include blue light which turns off melatonin production by the brain's pineal gland (recall, melatonin helps induce sleep). Blue light blocking glasses can help or apps that allow you to look at red light on the screen. Near infrared light may help too.
- Sleep in a dark, quiet, comfortable environment. If needed experiment with an eye mask, wax earplugs or noise preventing headphones. Look at red light rather than blue light screens before bed. Don't take your mobile phone to bed with you!
- Air and let light into your bedroom during the day. Keep a window slightly open at night if it is safe and comfortable to do so.
- Avoid overheating. It is best to sleep in a cool room as snuggling under the covers signals to the brain its sleep time.
- Pace enough activities during the day. Regularly pause and take three slow deep breaths (see Appendix 5). If you do not do enough physical activity (paced) during the daytime you may get a second wind, or an adrenaline rush before bed. People affected by ME/CFS describe this as going to bed 'tired and wired.' The following day they are 'crashed' and wake up exhausted. Learning the Rest/Activity Dance will help here and improve your HRV.

Further Tips

Before Bedtime Routine

- Ensure you have taken your regular medication and/or supplements before bed.

- Meditate, relax and wind down before bedtime for 20 min to an hour. If it helps, change into your PJ's in advance and heat up a wheat bag. Reduce or dim the lights in your house an hour before bedtime. Try playing a background black screen Youtube sleep music track e.g., https://www.youtube.com/watch?v=5dhxKwr6G5c This all helps to increase the parasympathetic tone, increase relaxation, reduce active thinking by the brain and reduce pain levels by increasing the body's endorphins. (See Appendix 5 & 6).
- A hug, massage, cuddle or sexual intimacy, if you have the energy for it, can be wonderfully settling.

Bedroom Preparation

- Darken the bedroom with blackout curtains or use a sleep mask at night. This helps the brain to produce the melatonin needed for sleep. In the morning, exposure to bright natural light or a seasonal affective disorder (SAD) light is helpful.
- Use earplugs or soundproofing for noise, or sleep in a different bedroom from a snoring partner or rambunctious pet.
- Make sure the bed is comfortable so that it cushions the body and prevents the worsening of pain. Most people prefer medium firmness in a bed with a pillow top or eggshell foam on top. If back or hip pain is an issue and you sleep on your side, you could try sleeping with a thin pillow placed between your knees.

If Unable to Sleep

- Pain can disrupt the process of falling asleep and there are many non-medication and medication based approaches that can help. Gentle stretching or massage may help and if muscle cramp is a big issue a small dose of magnesium orally or topically, rubbed into the muscle before bed may help. Herbal remedies at low doses, paracetamol or tiny doses of amitriptyline can help with easing pain and falling to sleep.
- If unable to sleep for more than half an hour after going to bed, do a gentle muscle relaxation starting with your toes and moving up towards your head, until the next 'train of sleepiness arrives' and takes you off to sleep. You don't have to stay alert to the moment of falling asleep; given the opportunity the body knows how to do it for you. You might like to remind yourself of this; "my body knows how to sleep. I don't have to 'do it'"
- If emotional distress is keeping you awake, then try the Soften and Flow exercise. (See Appendix 6)

- Writing/drawing/venting an uncensored page of your concerns during the day allows you to offload your stress onto the page and then to tear it up and toss it out. This gives the brain a chance to problem-solve solutions. (See Chapter 15, Defusing the Loop)
- Use meditation/relaxation recordings to help the brain to turn off and relax/restore the body or try light reading (a book in preference to a screen). Prayer helps some people. Whatever brings you peace and ease.
- Pace with rests as required throughout the day but, unless you simply must sleep, avoid napping past 3 pm because it interferes with night-time sleep.
- Hormonal changes in women can disrupt the sleep cycle especially the night before the period comes on and during menopause due to hot flushes. Be especially attentive to your sleep routine before your period and sleep a little cooler during menopause, a partially open window can help.
- Recall three pleasant experiences from the day, each night after you climb under the covers (e.g., a laugh, a bird's song, a thing of beauty) and hold an image or a feeling of one of these as you let yourself drift off with a smile of gratitude on your face.
- If you wake up to go to the toilet or settle a child or pet, keep the lights low or carry a dull torch so as not to enliven the brain. Try and recall, if not unpleasant, the most recent dream you were having so you can get back to it when you return to bed. The quicker you make it back to bed the more likely you are to go back into the same phase of sleep you arose from.
- Depression can cause early morning waking e.g., in bed and asleep by 10pm and wide wake between 2 and 4am. If this is happening regularly see your doctor.
- If you need to stay awake for an extended time before bed, you might not fall asleep easily. If so, you may have to wait for the sleep train to come around the tracks again. In this case, perhaps read or make yourself a comforting warm drink and retire to bed again when sleepiness returns.

Stimulants and Sleep Inducers

- Have a light snack or small, warm, nutritious drink before bed (unless you have reflux/heartburn in which case it is better not to have anything within a couple of hours of bed). Remember to take your medication.
- Avoid nicotine.

- Avoid alcohol and reduce or eliminate stimulants like caffeine-containing beverages (coffee/tea/energy drinks) and food, especially after 3 pm.
- Take calcium &/or magnesium remedies or medications before bedtime if needed. Drink non-caffeinated herbal teas e.g., chamomile, fennel or peppermint to help the body to relax.

Also see *https://sleepfoundation.org/ask-the-expert/sleep-hygiene*

Table 2 Winning Tips for Better Sleep

Chapter 7
Key Points

- ✓ Unrefreshing sleep is a feature of ME/CFS.
- ✓ Sleep disorders can occur with or mimic ME/CFS.
- ✓ If you find you are dosing off often during the day you may have a 50% chance of being diagnosed with a sleep disorder, such as Sleep Apnoea or Restless Legs. If so, you may need a referral from your GP to a Sleep Specialist Clinic for a complete overnight assessment.
- ✓ Consider purchasing a biofeedback system like the OURA ring you can wear overnight and upload to an APP the next day to assess your sleep patterns at home. This can also help to teach you how to actively relax and which things modify your sleep.
- ✓ If pain, itchy skin or a blocked nose are an issue you may also need to address this with your doctor.
- ✓ Institute a winning bedtime routine, starting with my 'Top Seven Tips' and consider the other suggestions (see Table 2 above) in future.

- ✓ A range of medications including Amitriptyline and natural sleep inducers, such as melatonin, can help. Just remember to start at a lower dose than most people and build up slowly, as people with ME/CFS often only require a quarter of the usual dose to start with.

Chapter 8

NUTRITIONAL WISDOM

"Eating healthy food fills your body with energy and nutrients. Imagine your cells smiling back at you and saying: "Thank you!"."
KAREN SALMANSOHN

Food is fundamental to our survival. It contains the building blocks of our bodies. To understand how ME/CFS (and health generally) might be affected by our diet, it is worth taking a step back.

In a big picture sense, the context in which our body's cells find themselves is reflected in the biochemical environment that bathes and literally feeds them. In other words, our healthy or unhealthy diet is what we are giving our body's cells on a microscopic level to work with.

In addition, many of our cells die and are replaced many times during our lifetime, providing ongoing opportunity to change the epigenetic pattern (See *A Doctor's Journey Back to Health, Ch 14)* they are expressing. In some regions, such as the lining of our mouth, stomach and nose, the turnover is rapid, occurring in a matter of days. In other areas, like our immune system, white blood cells are being turned over in days to weeks whilst our red blood cells are replaced four-monthly. Even our liver is replaced annually and our entire skeleton every decade.[1]

By changing our diet, the nutrient and chemical context that our cells find themselves in is altered, affecting the way they function. In addition, the process involved in the production of new cells, comes under this fresh influence. In these two ways, a body part's cells expressing a disease, like ME/CFS, can change to expressing health. As I've explained in my previous book, epigenetic research into Multiple Sclerosis (MS) confirms this potential.

So clearly on a basic biochemical level food is an essential ingredient for improving ME/CFS. But food is much more than this. It carries many meanings for us, whether they be social, cultural, comfort, likes/dislikes or part of our identity, food is often front and center. Changing our diet can therefore bring many challenges. Nonetheless, the effort can be extremely rewarding with evidence for the role of food in both health and disease promotion ever-growing. In terms of ME/CFS, research has yet to identify the ideal diet,[2] but what can be said is that around 50% of people with ME/CFS report having food intolerances,[3] whilst weight problems, either gain or loss, are very common and can create additional stress, depression and reduced self-worth. A lack of capacity to exercise in people with ME/CFS can undermine their efforts of losing excess kilos. Still, a positive effect of getting more in tune with your dietary needs is a stabilizing of weight and appetite.

Instinctive Eating

Where to begin? In their new book, *Eat Like the Animals*,[4] authors Professors David Raubenheimer and Stephen Simpson from the University of Sydney's Charles Perkins Centre and School of Life and Environmental Sciences, present a synthesis of more than two decades of research. They reveal the reasons a baboon, a cat and a locust instinctively know what to eat to exactly balance their nutritional needs. This is a basic ability many humans seem to have lost and yet can quickly regain.

In the following podcast: https://www.abc.net.au/radionational/programs/scienceshow/how-our-bodies-tell-us-what-to-eat/12582438 Professor Raubenheimer points out that research has uncovered taste receptors beyond our tongues and noses to lower regions in our gut and respiratory systems. **These receptors, if operating correctly, can guide us to the foods we really need to eat. He points out that animals possess five appetites – for protein, carbohydrate, fat, salt and calcium.**

In our natural state these five appetites would have led us to carefully select foods to fulfil our needs. This was discovered by a PhD student, Caley Johnson, who studied the food selections of a wild baboon called, Stella. Stella's diverse choice of foods over a one-month period revealed a very tight correlation between protein, fat and carbohydrate intake, regardless of the fact her diet altered daily.

Dr. Raubenheimer goes on to explain, "In natural food environments these appetites cooperate to help animals choose a balanced diet. Humans have this ability too, but the modern food environment is so altered that our appetites can no longer work together. Rather, they compete, each vying for its own nutrient. It is this competition that causes us to over-eat fats and carbs, leading to obesity and the serious diseases that come with it."

Their research has revealed that we seek out fats and carbs in our diet not because we have a greater appetite for these things but because protein is diluted in our modern food-chain. Protein, it turns out, is number one when it comes to our five appetites and we will eat until our appetite for it is satisfied. This explains why people on a high protein diet generally lose weight as their protein appetite will be rapidly satisfied and they'll consequently eat less calories overall.

As I will explain in the next chapter, high protein diets such as the Ketogenic diet fall into the category of 'therapeutic diets' that should not be maintained over the long term as they can have detrimental consequences. Eating an excess of protein can shorten telomere length (telomeres are the caps holding our 46 chromosomes in place within our cells) and other such biological processes that hasten ageing and allow disease to form prematurely in the body.[5]

Co-author Prof Simpson adds, "we have made low-protein processed foods (chips, biscuits cereals, sweets etc.) taste unnaturally good. We've diluted protein in the food supply with ultra-processed fats and carbs. We've also disconnected the brake on our appetite systems by decreasing dietary fibre."

This is perfect for getting us to eat more of the wrong stuff. This may assist the bottom line of processed food manufacturers and retailers who profit from our confused, overstimulated appetites, but is devastating for our health, our *bottom* line. Food cultures globally have been changed by aggressive marketing of these products.

The researcher's advice is to follow three principles:

1. Surround yourself with Whole foods

Foods such as nuts, fruits, vegetables, healthy oils, unrefined grains, pulses and moderate amounts of quality meats if you wish. "Avoid meals and snacks that are factory-produced (i.e., processed), or buy them sparingly," says Professor Raubenheimer.

We have this amazing appetite system and research is showing us that all other species have their own version. We can allow it to operate its own magic by presenting it with wholesome food options and limiting the processed options that trick its biological sensors. We can then, ultimately, learn to trust our own appetite.

2. Aim for balance

There are many nutritional philosophies slugging it out today. To me, guidance comes from the diets of long-lived societies, as I've discussed elsewhere.[6,7] These cultures and the research we do have, points towards eating as whole food a diet as we can, learning to embrace as many and as big a variety of vegies along the way.

So, cut out or reduce 'whites,' i.e., highly processed foods, rich in sugar, white flour, fat and excess salt and poor in fibre and nutrients.

3. Make it a habit

The natural world isn't born with an encyclopaedia of instructions as to what to eat. Researchers have studied creatures from slime molds to elephants and found the same inherent capacity to balance their diets. We have that inherent capacity too, it's just a matter of reminding our bodies.

Professor Raubenheimer adds that before long, eating an enjoyable healthy diet will become automatic. "It's like learning a sport, to play a musical instrument, or to drive an automobile: at first it takes concentration, consciously applying rules, rehearsing them, and unlearning bad habits. And then it becomes second nature," he says.

The low GI diet suggestions in the next chapter will help you to get started and find a better nutritional track. Our own experience (authors Steven & Tori) and that of many of our patients, as people who'd developed a 'sweet tooth', was when we cut refined sugar from our diet, we craved it for around two weeks and then were happy enough to have lower GI sweeteners (I'll explain this in the next chapter) such as stevia or a little fruit to satisfy any sweet urge. However, if we slipped up, we'd once again crave sugary sweets for another fortnight and need to consciously avoid them again! So now we just say no to sugary snacks and feel better for it.

Before we go into my specific dietary suggestions in the next chapter, let's begin with some general suggestions for people with ME/CFS (see Table 1).

> **Table 1 General Suggestions**
> - If possible, get carers, friends or family to assist with grocery shopping and meal preparation.
> - Share a meal with them if it lifts your spirits and they can do the washing up!
> - Consider home delivered groceries or meals and vegetables that are prewashed and chopped. If you can afford it or have access to home grown, organic or pesticide free vegetables and fruit, these are best. However snap frozen vegetables maintain good nutrition.
> - Stews and soups that can be cooked in large batches and frozen and/or vacuum sealed in meal or snack size portions make for easy low-prep meals. A Slow Cooker can be of great assistance here and is a worthwhile inexpensive investment.
> - Avoid large meals within 3 hours of bedtime.
> - Well cooked foods with small amounts of salad may be more digestible initially.
> - A dry mouth and lips mean you're thirsty. Drink plenty of filtered water outside of mealtimes. Aim to drink at least half an hour before or after meals so as not to dilute the digestive juices of the stomach. (Unless you have medications, digestive enzymes or supplements to swallow with your meal).

The Migrating Motor Complex (MMC)

When people with ME/CFS are not hungry it is often due to a slowing of their digestive

track. Everything slows down when we are not active. Strategies to move things along

can be helpful. These strategies are sometimes referred to as 'prokinetics.'

The gut produces a coordinated peristaltic wave called the Migrating Motor Complex or MMC. It is like a large broom sweeping the fibre and less digestible contents of your stomach and intestines down towards your colon. It's the loudest gurgle you'll hear just before you start getting hungry again. This wave stops as soon as we put food in our mouths, hence when you are hungry aim to eat enough calories in your mealtimes without overfilling your stomach and then allow 2 hours between meals or snacks to let the MMC do its thing.

If poor appetite is an issue for you, Table 2 has some suggestions.

Table 2 Suggestions for Improving Appetite
- If you have lost interest in food or have a weak digestive system, you could try waiting till you are hungry before eating or stimulating your appetite by drinking a warm glass of water (two thirds of a cup of cold water with a third of a cup of boiled water). To this you can add a ½ squeezed fresh lemon, slice of fresh ginger and or turmeric and/or a teaspoon of apple cider vinegar mixed in with it. These foods are prokinetic and assist with the movement of food through the small intestine.
- Drink a full glass of a prokinetic beverage soon after waking/rising in the morning and/or sip on it throughout the day and/or 5 to 30 minutes before meals. (experiment and see the timing that works best for you i.e., to make you feel hungry). Alternatively, ginger tea alone, with peppermint oil capsules (ask your pharmacist) or digestive enzymes may help. (I found digestive enzymes before or with meals a particularly helpful supplement that improved my appetite so that I gained much needed weight.)
- Become aware of what works best for you, for example, try eating smallish meals or just three meals a day. Most of my patients with ME/CFS found smaller frequent meals preferable.
- If you can, wait at least 2 hours (or as long as you feel able) between meals or snacks, as this allows the Migrating Motor Complex (MMC) to move food downwards from the stomach, further along the small intestine to the large intestine (colon). Movement improves energy.
- Relax and enjoy your food.
- Chew well.
- Practice stopping eating before you feel full (85% full is enough).
- Sip on digestive tea herbs like peppermint, ginger, fennel, chamomile, licorice
- If able, take a short walk or some standing activity to aid digestion after meals.

The Case for Buying Organic

The safest and healthiest thing to do is to eat as many good quality vegetables and fruits as you can. But do we need to buy organic vegetables and fruit? When all the research is tabulated, the experts tell us there is not enough difference in nutritional value, from an individual health point of view, to be of concern,[8] although some organic farms may show marked increases in nutritional value.[9] That said, research does confirm that you decrease your exposure to pesticides by eating organic foods ahead of conventional ones,[10] and that this is the most pressing reason people give for choosing organic produce.[11]

Pesticides have been shown to build up in the bodies of children eating conventional food and subsequently are shown to be eliminated from the bodies of these same children when they're placed on an exclusively organic diet.[12] The American Academy of Pediatrics acknowledged the potential advantage of organic foods, especially in very young children.[13] Parents obviously agree with this, as sales of organic baby food are one of the fastest-growing organic food items.[14]

Recently the once thought to be safe herbicide (weed killer), 'Round Up' (glyphosate) was found to be unsafe for adults when it was linked to causing the cancer, Non-Hodgkins Lymphoma.[15] In addition the neurological disorder, Parkinson's Disease, has been linked to pesticide accumulation.[16]

Still, nutrition is key, and fresh and snap frozen vegies are still much better than no vegies. So, my suggestion would be: the fresher the better, home-grown if possible, then organic produce if affordable and then non-organic. Check out your local Farmers Market too.

To Supplement or not to Supplement?

In Chapter 4 we looked at supplements that may help in managing ME/CFS. In terms of diet and adequate nutrition in general, let me present some current ideas and research.

Some nutritionists are of the opinion that due to diminished soil quality, the nutritional content of most fruit and vegetables we eat has decreased over the last 50 years. Supporting this assertion are the findings of a careful survey in the UK from the Marine Research Centre and Ministry of Agriculture. They compared 27 vegetables, 20 fruits and ten meats over 50 years. They showed average falls of 48% in calcium and 27% in iron content, with similar or greater losses for other minerals like copper or magnesium.[17,18]

So, does this mean we should all be taking vitamin and mineral supplements? The answer is not so simple. Taking more is not necessarily better. In addition, vitamins and minerals contained in food are supported and integrated by other compounds within the food. Let's take the example of an apple.

In his revealing book, *Whole - Rethinking the Science of Nutrition*,[19] T Colin Campbell highlights a landmark research study published in the journal, *Nature. In this article, researchers reported their analysis of the composition of 100g (half a cup) of apple.*[20] They discovered that this amount of apple produced an antioxidant effect equivalent to 1500 mg of pure vitamin C. However, when they looked at how much vitamin C was actually present in the apple sample, it amounted to just 5.7 mg!

It turns out there are hundreds if not thousands of other chemicals, some of whom were contributing to this vitamin C-like effect.[21] It is mind expanding to think of how all these chemicals may be interacting and working together, influencing thousands of biochemical reactions within our bodies, leading to the variety of benefits we subsequently receive from a simple bite of apple.

In an understated way, as is often the language of scientists, the researchers concluded, "that natural antioxidants from fresh fruit could be more effective than a dietary supplement (of vitamin C)."[22]

Chapter 8
Key Points

- ✓ Food provides the building blocks for our ever-changing body.
- ✓ This and our understanding of epigenetics (see *A Doctor's Journey Back to Health. Ch 14*) provides us with an opportunity to improve our ME/CFS through our diet.
- ✓ We can relearn, like other animals, to eat instinctively again. (see *Eat Like the Animals*)
- ✓ General suggestions are given in Tables 1 and 2.
- ✓ Whole foods with plenty of vegies for various beneficial reasons.
- ✓ Promoting healthy soil regeneration is crucial for healthier people.
- ✓ Whole foods are more nutritious and cannot be fully replaced by vitamin supplements.

Chapter 9
LOW GI DIET AND MINI FASTS

"Let medicine be thy food and food be thy medicine."
HIPPOCRATES

"If you keep good food in your fridge, you will eat good food."
ERRICK MCADAMS

In this chapter I'll share with you the specific diet I employed personally, clinically and successfully with many of my patients. It is in effect a 'training wheels' diet that ultimately leads to the 'instinctive eating' diet we explored in the previous chapter. We will also look at how taking breaks in our eating, i.e., a mini-fast, may rejig our health for the good.

Fad, Therapeutic and Maintenance Diets

From a treatment perspective, diets can be broadly placed along a spectrum from **fad** to **therapeutic** to **maintenance**. At one end of the spectrum, **fad** diets like the 1970's Israeli Army Diet or the Grapefruit diet fit into the category of Very Low-Calorie diets specifically designed for rapid weight loss. They are often low fat and high GI (I'll explain this below) and can vary from profoundly dangerous to beneficial in the short term but nutrient deficient and therefore unsafe in the long term. They might help Cinderella fit into her ball gown but after midnight, the rebound weight gain begins!

Therapeutic diets, such as a fresh juice fast, the FODMAP diet[1] or the very-low carb Keto diet, have a broader therapeutic intention in mind to allay gut problems and/or generally improve health. These diets may be beneficial in the short to medium-term but not healthy to continue in the long-term either. They also lack some essential nutrients and importantly lack fiber, more on this in a moment.

At the other end of the spectrum, **maintenance** diets like the Mediterranean diet,[2] which has been more extensively studied than any other healthy human diet, can be safely continued indefinitely and will assist in maintaining health.

No single diet applies to everyone as different illnesses, body-types, food allergies and intolerances mean a diet might require specific tweaking to bring about the best health outcomes. Nonetheless, there are common issues that people with ME/CFS need to address.

Food Allergies and Intolerances

Food allergies and/or intolerances are a growing problem. As mentioned earlier, around 50% of people with ME/CFS report food intolerances.[3] If this applies to you, then you may need to modify the dietary suggestions I have made thus far. Consulting an allergist/nutritionist/dietician/naturopath with a special interest in managing food intolerances would be a good idea.

For instance, some people find removing any combination of wheat, dairy, eggs, sugar, soy, gluten and/or grains from their diet improves their symptoms, energy and mental clarity in particular. Others, particularly those overweight, have found benefit from the Paleo or Ketogenic (Keto) diets.[4,5] The Keto diet is particularly effective at improving brain fog, and inducing weight loss if this is suitable for your situation, but beware the lack of fiber.[6] Again, I would caution going beyond a few months on these low carb therapeutic diets. Even the well-researched and medically accepted for IBS, FODMAP diet, has been shown to cause nutritional deficiencies if used beyond three months.[7] Hence, if you are interested in looking into these diets, I recommend doing so under supervision from an experienced health practitioner familiar with these programs.

There is, however, a diet that you can safely try now, a low Glycemic Index (GI) diet.

A Whole Food Low GI Diet

The Glycaemic Index (GI) is a value from 100 to 1, assigned to carbohydrate foods - like bread, rice, cereals, potatoes, desserts, sugar etc.- where glucose is the maximum at 100 and all other carbohydrate foods are ranked according to how slowly or how quickly these foods cause increases in blood glucose ("sugar") levels after we swallow them.[8]

As carbohydrate food is broken down and absorbed into the blood stream from the gut, blood glucose levels rise, ingested pure glucose is therefore the fastest. This triggers the hormone insulin to be released into the bloodstream from the pancreas gland. Insulin then assists in moving this glucose from inside the blood vessels into the body's cells, where it is used within the cell for energy production. The GI therefore provides a relative ranking of carbohydrate in foods according to how rapidly they affect blood glucose levels and insulin release.

Many people with ME/CFS find high GI carbohydrate foods give them a brief energy pick me up followed by a significant energy crash. This is because the high GI foods trigger surges in insulin and thus rapid changes in blood glucose levels. In contrast, carbohydrates with a low GI value (55 or less, see Table 1) are more slowly digested, absorbed and metabolized and cause a lower, slower more even rise in blood glucose and insulin levels.[9]

Table 1 Glycaemic Index (GI) Food Sample		
Glucose = 100	Potato boiled 78	cow's milk full cream 39
White bread 75	potato instant mash 87	soy milk 34
Multigrain bread 53	banana 51	rice milk 86
Rolled oat porridge 55	orange juice fresh 50	chickpeas 32
Instant oat porridge 79	apple unpeeled 36	lentils 28
For further examples see: https://www.health.harvard.edu/diseases-and-conditions/glycemic-index-and-glycemic-load-for-100-foods)		

People with ME/CFS that I consulted with were provided with the low Glycemic Index (GI) dietary suggestions in APPENDIX 4 as a starting point. It is similar to the diet recommended by the Austin Hospital's ME/CFS program in Melbourne. This diet aims to keep blood sugar (glucose) levels as even as possible throughout the day. Thus, fast release refined, processed and sugary foods are avoided, and this reduces insulin surges and blood sugar swings which, as I've said, can contribute to energy crashes.

Hence, foods or food combinations with a low Glycemic Index (low GI) are the ideal. By eating high-fiber carb-foods as well as combining these with protein and healthy fat can assist this process, as they slow down the absorption from the gut into the bloodstream. A good starting point is to eliminate all the whites from your diet: white bread, white rice, white flour, potatoes, and sugar.

Note, in Table 1 how the level of food processing effects the foods GI. For example, porridge made with whole rolled oats (55) versus instant oats (79).

I have outlined more specific dietary tips in APPENDIX 4 - Low GI Diet Suggestions.

Note that white meats are some of the highest protein foods and are not in the list of things to eliminate from your diet unless you are vegetarian.

Diet and Dysbiosis ? A Cause

There is evidence that people affected by ME/CFS have an unhealthy balance of bowel bugs (dysbiosis) with less variety when compared with healthy people.[10] The importance of a healthy gut microbiome (population of bugs) in achieving good health is becoming increasingly recognized for a wide range of illnesses.[11,12] Evidence that altering this for the better can improve ME/CFS is found in research that showed that fecal microbial transplant (inserting healthy poo, with its trillions of beneficial bacteria, from a healthy donor into the bowel of a person with ME/CFS) can benefit some people, maybe up to half, with ME/CFS.[13]

Another study found that people affected by ME/CFS who took a particular probiotic (Lactobacillus casei strain Shirota), after two months experienced significantly less anxiety than those who took placebo.[14] Dysbiosis has also been implicated as a possible cause of Irritable Bowel Syndrome, a common co-existing problem amongst people with ME/CFS.

The gut-brain connection is being increasingly acknowledged. For instance, in other neurological disorders such as Parkinson's Disease (PD) where the neurotoxin alpha synuclein, found in the brain cells of people with PD, has been located in the nervous system surrounding the gut and has been shown to travel upwards from there via the vagus nerve to the brain.[15] Perhaps this is how Parkinson's begins. There have also been some positive results in treating PD with long wavelength near infrared light applied externally to the abdomen, which has been demonstrated to not only change the colons microbiome (photobiomodulation), but improve Parkinson's symptoms.[16] A low carbohydrate diet has also helped, but it is early days in terms of the research.[17]

It's likely we'll find the gut microbiome to be important in the origin and treatment of ME/CFS too, and we don't need to wait until this is confirmed to act on this.

The Fiber Key

In the previous chapter we looked at Professors Raubenheimer and Simpson's suggestion that we encourage good bacteria in our gut by eating as close to a whole food (unprocessed) plant-based diet as possible, with lots of fiber in the form of vegetables, fruit, nuts and seeds. Plant fiber and resistant starch are the best foods for the helpful bacteria in the gut.

One of the most researched beneficial fibers is pectin, a water-soluble fiber found in a wide range of fruits and vegie. Examples include: apples (with the skin), citrus peel, sweet potato, green beans and pumpkin. For a fuller list see

https://www.livestrong.com/article/289067-list-of-foods-high-in-pectin/

So, it may well be true that 'an apple a day keeps the doctor away.'[18]

If you are not used to eating a lot of fiber or resistant starch, it may cause some additional bloating and flatulence, so it is best then to build up your fiber intake gradually over several months. Pre-soaking of, for example, chia seeds or porridge oats in water overnight in the fridge before draining, rinsing and cooking can help digestibility and be gentler on the stomach too. Legumes, nuts and seeds can also be made more digestible by presoaking in water overnight in the fridge.

A little cultured food with each meal (like sauerkraut, kefir, yoghurt, miso or kimchee) can help digestion too, but like fiber can cause abdominal discomfort and bloating if introduced too quickly. So once again you'll need to see what works best for you. Introduce new things one at a time so you can tell what's best.

If present, treatment of irritable bowel syndrome (IBS) with the low FODMAP diet helps some patients, as it did with Katie (See Chapter 14). Some people with ME/CFS have small intestinal bacterial overgrowth (SIBO) and/or leaky gut and have developed new food sensitivities/intolerances. In these people, prokinetic treatments that help to keep the Migrating Motor Complex (MMC) moving the digested food along (see Table 2 previous chapter), can make a big difference.[19]

Reducing and avoiding sensitive foods which worsen symptoms can be helpful. For example, you could rotate your foods (especially carbohydrates like wheat, oats or quinoa) every 4–5 days so you avoid developing sensitivities. If intestinal dysbiosis is present people may also improve their symptoms by taking L-glutamine or butyrate and/or by using probiotics proven to help IBS. Be aware that not all probiotics are the same; choose one with at least one research study showing its effectiveness in IBS. A PubMed search at: https://www.ncbi.nlm.nih.gov/pubmed/ may help you find one you could try or ask your GP or chemist. Even so, some 'take it and see' may be needed to find the right one for you.

A Special Case for treating Constipation

Many of the patients I saw, myself included, had problems with constipation. Being sedentary, as imposed by the illness, increases the likelihood of constipation developing. Dealing with constipation can free up energy, reduce malaise and myalgia (muscle pain) and improve mood. I found that a daily dose of psyllium husks 2 heaped teaspoons twice daily, well stirred into a full glass of warm water helpful. Increasing my water intake generally, having sufficient fiber in my diet and using occasional glycerol suppositories if 'bunged up' were all helpful. I also became very comfortable using a rectal enema or syringe with plain warmish water on occasion. Ask your pharmacist to order in a rectal enema kit for you.

Intermittent Mini Fasts for Health

Fasting to reboot our bodies back towards health has a long history. Human research into its health benefits is in its early stages but is promising.[20,21] Bear in mind that I am discussing mini fasting in this instance and am not recommending long periods of fasting for people with ME/CFS. I am unaware of any research involving fasting and people with ME/CFS, but I have read anecdotal reports of it being very helpful and can only echo this from my personal experience. Given that it's free and has a long record of usefulness generally, I believe it is worth exploring.

For many people with ME/CFS, particularly those who are underweight as I was, it is difficult for them to fast as blood insulin and glucose levels can fluctuate widely, requiring regular intake of food to quell the associated energy dips. So, my suggestion would be to spend at least two months sticking to a low GI diet, stabilizing insulin and glucose levels, aiming to reach a **2-hour break once per day** between food intake to activate the Migrating Motor Complex (MMC) before attempting longer mini-fasts. Even one 2-hour break from eating during the day can help a delicate digestive system to rebalance.

Keep in mind that in this instance we are not aiming to fast to achieve weight loss. Nor are we going to deny adequate nutrition, we are performing it as a therapy, giving the body's clean-up crew a chance

CHAPTER 9 LOW GI DIET AND MINI FASTS

to detoxify and rejuvenate itself, a process known as **autophagy**. This can result in improved energy levels and clearer thinking, therefore assisting with brain fog.

Once you have conquered the 2-hour between meals/snacks mini-fasts, I suggest you start a program of longer overnight mini-fasts by leaving at least **eight hours** in which you refrain from eating food (you can drink as much water or herbal teas as you wish). Do this fast from say 10pm till 6am where hopefully most of the time will be spent asleep. Most people with ME/CFS can manage this without crashing. If not, then you can try to build up to it using the low GI diet (see Appendix 4) for another month or more and once again try not snacking between meals, so you get at least two two-hour fasts during the day, only eating when you feel hungry. If you are already underweight and lose more weight you may have to rethink your strategy. I found these mini fasts improved my appetite so that I ultimately gained much needed weight as I became hungrier and was able to eat more after two hours of not eating.

Once you are happy you can do an overnight eight-hour fast, then you can try a **12 hour fast**, from say 7pm to 7am. Again, most of the fast will still happen overnight and my experience is that people may feel hungry in the evening, but this usually settles with a glass of water, a herbal or green tea and distraction. Failing this, a spoon full of coconut oil, olive oil, butter or any fat should safely quell the hunger without disrupting the benefits of the fast.

Once you go to bed your hunger will settle. In this instance the hunger is a positive sign that the body is doing internal housework and you can reassure yourself that you will be well fed in the morning. Try and do this once or twice a week. (You can safely do it more often if it feels beneficial and you are not losing weight).

Knowing the hunger will disappear overnight and that you will be eating in the morning, **aim to make hunger your friend.** After all, it is the messenger that health restoration is underway in your body.

To this end, once again, reassure yourself that you will not miss out on food, just have it between different hours of the day. You might then timetable a 12 hour fast once or twice a week. If this is working for you, you can introduce this pattern of eating with 8 to 12 hour fasts most weeks. It can be very healing (See Table 2).[22] Beyond this I would not recommend longer fasting for people with ME/CFS unless recommended and supervised by your doctor.

If you're interested in reading more about this topic, the person I'm aware most widely published on the health effects of fasting is Professor Valter Longo at the University of Southern California. His website is: https://www.valterlongo.com/

If you're interested in more directions and information about fasting with ME/CFS, I encourage you to work closely with a nutritionist or clinician who is familiar with intermittent fasting. In the meantime, here is a link to an excellent website and blog where a health practitioner, Dr Courtney Craig puts her own recovery from ME/CFS down to, at least in part, incorporating intermittent fasting into her life (see link below).

https://www.healthrising.org/blog/2014/07/10/craig-fasting-health-fibromyalgia-chronic-fatigue-syndrome/

Table 2 Potential Health Benefits of Fasting

1. Improves blood glucose control
2. Anti-inflammatory
3. Heart health – may improve blood pressure, cholesterol and triglycerides
4. Brain function improved
5. Weight loss/metabolism booster
6. Muscle strength improved
7. Delayed ageing
8. Cancer prevention

See *https://www.healthline.com/nutrition/fasting-benefits#section1*

CHAPTER 9 LOW GI DIET AND MINI FASTS

**Chapter 9
Key Points**

- ✓ Your diet is very important. It can improve your health or make it worse.
- ✓ We do not have enough research at this stage to advise the best diet for ME/CFS but cutting out white high GI foods is a safe healthy way to begin.
- ✓ Your first priority is making sure you can provide yourself with enough healthy food for adequate nutrition. Ask for help if you need it (friends, family, GP, dietician/nutritionist, support group).
- ✓ If you wish to try an approach, a whole (unprocessed) low GI diet with lots of veggies, allowing 2 hours between meals or snacks if you can, is a good place to start (see Appendix 4).
- ✓ Fasting has a long history of health benefits. Hence you may wish to try rejigging your epigenetics with the mini fasts I describe in this chapter. A two hour fast alone allows the Migrating Motor Complex (MMC) to activate more easily which can improve well-being.

Chapter 10
PACING AND THE ENERGY ENVELOPE

"...you must always be yourself and do things at your own pace. Someday, you'll catch up."
NATSUKI TAKAYA (JAPANESE MANGA ARTIST)

"Hamba gashle" - Make haste slowly.
ZULU SAYING

Most people with ME/CFS, including myself, were healthy and fit at one time in their lives. Because of this, the whole idea of pacing one's day can seem ridiculous. Most of you will remember days when you expended energy on lots of physical and mental activity, had a good eight or nine hours sleep and woke up refreshed and restored, ready to go again. If you have been healthy in this way you can see how having to pace yourself feels unnecessary and constraining.

However, when one has ME/CFS, the constraints that are placed upon us by the illness are so severe that if we are to escape from the low-energy realm we find ourselves in, we must learn to conserve what we have so that our body can use some of the reserved energy for healing. From this position we can steadily launch our bid for a better life.

For people with ME/CFS who are not bedbound, there is often a 'boom and bust' lifestyle which is characterized by activity peaks followed by long periods of rest. Being unaware of our body's signals for rest and pushing on regardless can trigger ME/CFS relapses and for some may have triggered the onset of the illness to start with,[1,2] e.g., athletes who overtrain.

Let me emphasize here that not everyone with this pattern of behavior will end up with ME/CFS, however, some people who do not learn how to pace their activity with adequate rest may develop other physical or mental health problems. So pacing is becoming an essential skill in this modern world.

For those of us with ME/CFS a modification in how we live our day to day lives will be vital if we are to have **any** chance of breaking free of it or at least managing it in a way that gives us a life back. Maintaining a pattern of boom and bust just ain't gonna cut it!

A Cautionary Tale - Caitlin's Crash

You might recall meeting Caitlin in Chapter 6. Caitlin, 43, married with two young sons, had meningitis and had gone on to develop ME/CFS following this episode. As part of assisting Caitlin I introduced her early on to a Defusing the Loop technique. I won't go into details now as we will look at mind-body approaches in more detail in Chapter 15. I will say, however, that what happened next delighted and then shocked me. In fact, it changed the way I approached my patients with ME/CFS from then on.

At the time I did not realize just how critical it would be to teach Caitlin about pacing before unleashing the liberation of energy that can sometimes occur with a specifically targeted ME/CFS mind-body technique. What delighted me was that during and immediately after teaching Caitlin this technique she felt her anxieties melt away and new energy filter in. What shocked me came to light at our next consultation. Caitlin had gone home and over the next five days proceeded to expend more physical and mental energy than she had done in years. This included a daily equivalent of briskly walking several kilometres, doing her grocery shopping, catching up for coffee with friends and then picking her kids up from school. Prior to this, most of her days were spent resting on the couch.

When she returned for our scheduled follow-up two weeks later, she was a wreck. She related to me that after five-days of frenetic activity she had crashed badly. Her muscle pain was severe, she was sleeping very poorly at night and was sleeping a further two hours during the day. It would take Caitlin a further month before she would return to the same level of energy she'd had, prior to me introducing this mind-body technique.

I've not included this story to frighten you, but rather to emphasize the point that if you wish to take on any new strategy that may improve your energy levels it is best to learn the principles and practices of pacing first. The harsh truth is, without incorporating pacing, you will most likely continue to crash and burn consistently and never learn how to maximize your capacities and give yourself a chance to restore much of your life.

"But I Can't Pace – It makes me anxious and it's boring. It's just not my personality!"

I heard this statement often in our clinic. If this is what you're telling yourself about pacing, there are seven points I'd like to make:

1. What you are telling yourself is a limiting belief system not a truth. Pacing, like walking, playing golf or knitting is something we can all learn. You may not like it or be the best in the world at it, but ***you can do it***. I'm not just saying this either, this has been proven by research.[3] As I mentioned in the introduction the brain forms new pathways in response to repetition, this is called neuroplasticity. Just like a determined 74-year old grandma who has never played golf can learn how to play with regular practice, so you *can* learn

to pace. The less you use the boom bust superhighways (i.e., nerve pathways) dominating a part of your brain now, the more they will fade and will be replaced by pacing ability pathways.

2. Pacing may feel strange and constricting for the first few months. However, in time it will become an enjoyable dance allowing you to achieve and appreciate more activities in your day, not less. You'll also receive more rejuvenation from your rest periods. In the context of your lifespan the discomfort of the first few months will be inconsequential compared to the benefits you will receive.

3. Saying this, some people, like I was, are extremely driven on the inside. Their inner drive is a positive attribute on the one hand and allows them to achieve a great deal in life, but it can also be a negative attribute, one which if left unchecked can keep sabotaging our progress. If you relate to this description, you may need to go to Chapter 15 and see if the strategies taught there might help.

4. If severe anxiety is present this can cause a drain in your energy without accomplishing any activity at all and it's wise to take this into account, especially if the activities you are planning to accomplish are likely to provoke further anxiety. Pacing alone is a good strategy to reduce anxiety as you can tell yourself that you will rest after a certain amount of time. If anxiety is still a big issue you may find that once you've mastered the basics of pacing along with the active rest and defusing strategies taught in Chapters 13 and 15, the anxiety will reduce and ease will grow.

5. There are also good free online mental health support sites such as https://www.mentalhealthonline.org.au/, an Australian government supported initiative, to help to

address anxiety using Cognitive Behavioral Therapy (CBT). Beyond this, as I mention in Chapter 15, some people have deeper issues and seeking further psychotherapeutic help with a psychologist or counsellor may be beneficial too, if you are well enough to access them.

6. You may require medication or a natural therapy, at least for a few weeks, to reduce your anxiety to allow you to build your skills in anxiety reduction, so you can have a go at this program. CBD oil maybe worth trying (See Chapter 4).

7. Even if you still think pacing is not for you, your body *is already* pacing you in the form of 'crash days' and a perpetual 'Ground Hog Day.' I'm just reminding you that you can break this pattern and try another way. Just commit to six weeks and see how you go. Rest assured the boom and bust way will be waiting for you if you choose to go back to it.

Why bother? What research says - The Energy Envelope Theory

The Energy Envelope Theory for managing ME/CFS recommends that people affected by this disease pace their activity according to their available energy resources.[4,5] In this approach, the phrase, 'staying within the envelope,' is used to designate a comfortable range of energy use in which you avoid both over-exertion and under-exertion, maintaining a healthier equilibrium of activity over time.

Many people with ME/CFS need to be encouraged to do less in order to decrease the discrepancy between perceived and expended energy. Others need to be encouraged to increase their activity if they have the appropriate amount of perceived energy to do so. The key is to not consistently over-expend energy supplies thereby depleting the 'envelope' of available energy. Rather than a cure, this approach focuses on improving the ability of people affected by ME/CFS to become more self-aware, so they can reduce energy crashes and cope with their illness better. It can, though, do much more than this.

Research involving 81 people affected by ME/CFS, looked at the health effects of teaching this energy management approach. It found that 49 out of the 81 people succeeded in keeping expended energy close to self-rated available energy (i.e., through their own estimates they were able to stay within their own energy envelope). When followed up, those 49 people had significant improvements in physical functioning and fatigue 12 months later.[6]

The Out of 100 Envelope Technique

One simple lesson you can learn from this research is that you can hone your own skills of self-awareness. Just like the participants in the study, you can estimate at the beginning of each day your perceived energy availability for that day out of 100 units (where 100 is having as much energy as you had when you were completely healthy). You then compare that with the amount of energy you feel you expended that day at day's end also out of 100.

For example, on one particular day you might come up with an estimate of 30 units of energy available in your envelope that morning. If by days end you estimate an expended energy of 20, this indicates you were within your energy envelope and that you could have included a little more activity utilizing up to 10 more units that day. By contrast you might have estimated 30 units at the start of the day and end the day feeling that you had utilized 40 units. It is likely that you will experience a depletion of your energy in subsequent days and need a greater amount of rest to redress the shortfall.

You might be surprised how this simple technique can restore more trust between you and your body. As you learn to self-monitor (without judgement) and begin to self-regulate with more confidence, your energy expenditure will more naturally come to match your capacity more often.

Pacing

Another effective and slightly different way of doing this is by pacing. Both methods can be used together complimenting each other. The difference being that pacing involves more moment by moment energy availability check-ins, not just at the beginning and end of the day. The aim here is to be as active as you are able within the limits imposed by the illness,[7,8] ignoring symptoms that do not make you feel unwell, but **either resting or changing** to an activity involving different muscles when more serious symptoms occur, indicating that your 'limits' have been exceeded (e.g., onset of muscle pain, dizziness/faint, brain fog).[9]

Goudsmit and her colleagues[10] used pacing as part of a multi-component ME/CFS program with very low side effect rates. Their physician-led program found significant differences between the people with ME/CFS treated in this way and controls (those not given the program) for fatigue, bodily symptoms, and self-efficacy. In addition, using this approach, improvements were maintained at the 12-month follow-up, suggesting the skills learnt had a long-term benefit. This long-term benefit is quite unusual in behaviour change research and is usually indicative of how much better people with ME/CFS were feeling while pacing their day in this way. This confirms my experience that people with ME/CFS are highly motivated to get well and if given a way to do this, can.

Invoking both energy envelope and pacing ideas involves mindfully tuning into your energy levels and becoming more self-aware, so that you break up activities before you become overly tired. This may not be an issue if you have 100 units of energy to use within a given day. But if you have ME/CFS and only 10 units are available, you need to use these wisely. You can think of it like budgeting, tune into how much energy you feel you have to spend, rest when needed and budget activities accordingly. It is important to remember not to be underactive or overactive but aim to use the energy available. Staying within your available energy envelope increases the opportunity for building your energy bank account and can move you towards better health.

For example, for someone with moderate ME/CFS who estimates they have 15 units of available energy that day, standing up at the sink washing dishes for 10 minutes un-paced, could, say, use 5 units of energy, leaving only 10 units to get through the rest of the day. If instead, at the moment they notice the onset of muscle pain and fatigue six minutes in, they stop and put their feet up for five minutes before returning for another short stint, they could still have their 15 units available for the rest of the day. The rest breaks in between activity or simply varying activities, for example (again in mild to moderate CFS) sitting down and paying your bills before returning to the washing-up, can restore or maintain energy.

In my experience, this is enhanced and even more restorative if the break involves mindful relaxation, such as slow deep breathing, focusing on the feeling of the breath flowing slowly in and slowly out (see Appendix 5). Mindful relaxation can have profound effects in people living with severe ME/CFS as well. We will look at some simple techniques, some taking just 30 seconds, in Chapter 13. This is a proactive step on from pacing; what I call 'the rest activity dance' and I'll explore this in more detail with you in chapters 13 and 14.

The downside to this is that activities take longer to complete, and people often find this frustrating to begin with. This period of frustration is worse in the initial six to eight weeks and if you can get through this short time you can begin to build up to more activity and less rest and in so doing, find you're able to resume more participation in daily life.

Philosophy

Philosophically, applying this approach as an ME/CFS rehabilitation management tool involves a shift in attitude for many people, namely, accepting and working within the limits imposed by the illness rather than fighting against them and pushing through. But don't be fooled, this is not a passive approach, it involves skillful monitoring of day-to-day choices and self-regulation. Within the area of rehabilitation of chronic illnesses, this approach has some similarities to Acceptance and Commitment therapy, which emphasizes acceptance and commitment along with behavior-change strategies.[11]

Research confirms that by just using this Energy Envelope Theory and Pacing conservation approach alone, over time, people affected by ME/CFS can find that they experience fewer crashes and decreased fatigue and symptom severity.[12]

Note: There are online ME/CFS websites teaching Envelope Theory and Pacing and I encourage you to spend some well-paced time learning and/or re-learning this critical skill – see:

https://emerge.org.au/diagnosis/managing-symptoms-daily-basis/pacing/#.Xdo0KdVS8dc

http://www.cfidsselfhelp.org/library/managing-your-energy-envelope

Re-challenging

Re-challenging with a new activity, like say a two minute phone chat, once a week is a positive way to begin to expand what has become, after a minimum of six months of debility (three months in children), a contracted existence for many. It's a bit like reclaiming land after a high tide. It's like ME/CFS has come through and washed away huge chunks of your life. Re-challenging does not have to be with a big activity either; it will depend on where you are at. It might start with wriggling your toes in bed and or rolling over in bed, as Samantha Miller did (see Ch 11) as her initial recovery step. For others it may be sitting up on the side of your bed for 30 seconds or sitting outside in the fresh air for a few minutes.

People with less severe ME/CFS might like to try a five-minute phone call, or if you're up to it, going out for a coffee for 20 or 30 minutes. In this instance you might decide to involve the other person by getting them to act as a timer. As I said, in time you'll not need to be as rigid timewise but at least for the first 3 to 6 months stick with it.

Be sure to make it **fun** too! Come up with a list of things you think you can manage and pluck one out each week. For example, you could put all your ideas on a page then cut them out and pace them in a hat ready for the 'Monday Plucking Ceremony.'

The good news is you don't have to be in great shape to begin this life affirming process, just think of something manageable that you haven't done since being unwell, budget some available energy for it that week and do it. As you gain in confidence, longer term goals will look more possible. As Ruth found, in the long run this might even build to an activity like online part-time study or work.

Chapter 10
Key Points

- ✓ Like reading or writing, pacing for people with ME/CFS is an essential skill we can all learn. I've outlined a way to introduce this and there are also directions to free or inexpensive online courses that can teach you pacing.
- ✓ As neuroplasticity suggests, the more you practice, the healthier the nerve pathways you'll build.
- ✓ As most people with ME/CFS discover, not learning to pace within your energy envelope leads to endless cycles of suffering with Post Exertional Malaise (PEM). This boom/bust pattern is reversed through pacing, a fact proven by researchers.
- ✓ Even if you are resting during the day, this does not mean you're pacing well if you then go and overexert yourself or not exert yourself at all.
- ✓ If you stick with this pacing approach avoiding PEM for 6 to 8 weeks, then you'll be well on your way to a better life.
- ✓ Re-challenging with a new activity a week, which can be as simple as sitting on the edge of your bed or outside in a garden for 30 seconds, can build confidence and be a positive affirmation, that despite the illness, you can still choose to participate in life in simple yet appreciative ways.

Chapter 11
THE ART OF MICRO-REHAB

*"It is not enough to climb the tree,
we must be able to get down too."*
TKV DESIKACHAR (YOGA TEACHER)

*"You must find a way to exercise safely.
If you do not exercise you will get worst."*
**DR NANCY KLIMAS,
LEADING ME/CFS RESEARCHER AND CLINICIAN FLORIDA, US**

The great paradox with ME/CFS is that overexertion worsens the condition whilst the right amount of activity can improve it. In order to restore stamina, you need to find a way to safely increase movement. Even if you are experiencing a relapse with Post Exertional Malaise (PEM), you can still move a little. Unfortunately, many people with ME/CFS who consulted with me, had reached a point where PEM meant, Post **Exercise** (instead of Exertional) Malaise. In other words, they'd become so fearful of exercise they avoided it altogether!

Make no mistake, as Dr Klimas's quote suggests above, underdoing it is as dangerous a recipe as overdoing it. It can be challenging though, so in the next three chapters we will unveil some of the secrets to getting it right.

Hormesis

The overarching concept of hormesis applies here, **appropriate challenge builds strength**. To begin, the challenge is to find the right starting amount of rehabilitation activity and very gradually introduce more physical movement from there. Best to start this exploration when you are not experiencing a PEM relapse.

If done right, apart from its beneficial impact on ME/CFS symptoms, all of which can improve, it can start to increase stamina. It is also an essential step in restoring a deconditioned body (loss of muscle mass and bone density that occurs through prolonged inactivity).

Can we Rehabilitate 'sick' Mitochondria?

In my earlier book, *A Doctor's Journey Back to Health Chapter 10*, we discovered research that demonstrated people with ME/CFS have a problem within their mitochondria ('energy batteries') within each body cell. This means aerobic exercise capacity is affected so that anaerobic metabolism is recruited more quickly than in healthy people to create energy.[1,2]

In addition, the immune system responds differently to maximal exercise efforts than that of sedentary people given the same task, especially if repeated 24 hours later.[3,4] This seems to be caused by the release of chemicals known as cytokines triggered by overexertion.

It is also worth repeating that the blood concentration levels and patterns of these chemical cytokines can accurately predict the level of debility being experienced by the person with ME/CFS, confirming a real physical problem is at work here.[5] Hence, the need to avoid, if possible, overexertion and its result, PEM.

It is also why it was suggested to rename ME/CFS in 2015 as Systemic Exertion Intolerance Disease (SEID) as no other disease we know of creates this response.[6] Twenty-three studies had confirmed this abnormal cytokine response when maximal exertion was performed on two consecutive days.[7] Critically, however, this does not mean people with ME/CFS should avoid exercise all together, but rather to do what

CHAPTER 11 THE ART OF MICRO-REHAB

can be **easily** managed (i.e., well below maximal) and slowly build from there.

More recently the discovery of the autonomic nervous system abnormality known as Chronotropic Intolerance (CI), a sluggish heart rate increase in response to exertion, has helped us to understand and design safer rehab approaches.

> The World Health Organization (WHO) defines rehabilitation as: "a set of interventions needed when a person is experiencing or is likely to experience limitations in everyday functioning due to ageing or a health condition, including chronic diseases or disorders, injuries or traumas. Examples of limitations in functioning are difficulties in thinking, seeing, hearing, communicating, moving around, having relationships or keeping a job."[8]
>
> Exercise is defined by the Cambridge Dictionary as: "physical activity that you do to make your body strong and healthy."[9] In clinical research circles exercise is simply defined as time set aside for a specific physical activity. In truth, for people with ME/CFS all activity i.e., activities of daily living (ADL'S) can feel like exercise. Going to the toilet, showering, washing the dishes, making the bed etc. So, let's be clear, the approach we'll be exploring in the next few chapters is placing exercise in the service of restoring function, i.e., rehabilitation, so that life in general can become more expansive and enjoyable.

After my brain surgery for Parkinson's Disease in December 2018, in which two probes were inserted into my brain and attached to a stimulator under my skin, much like a heart pacemaker, I was eventually transferred to a Rehabilitation ward where I started my rehab. This involved two weeks as an inpatient working on my balance, strength and ability to walk again. In the physio 'Gym' with me at that time was Charlie, a young man 23 years of age who'd come off his motorbike at 80km/hr and was recovering from multiple fractures, including a fractured pelvis.

Given I'd been wheelchair bound for the previous five years, strengthening muscles and rewiring new pathways in response to repetition (i.e., neuroplasticity) so that I could walk upright again was daunting. But watching Charlie barely able to stand aided by his physio was humbling. We were both motivated though, and worked hard within our own limitations, limitations that continued to expand with each session. During our one-hour program we would rest as needed, drink water smile at each other, then carry on. After each session I would be returned to my hospital room in a wheelchair where I would rest, often sleeping for an hour or so.

At the end of each week the physios would test us with a six-minute walk test. I would walk back and forth along a 10-metre runway, stopping and resting as much as I needed, for 6 minutes. By fortnights end I was able to walk unaided for 130 meters needing to rest three times over 6 minutes. Holding onto parallel bars, Charlie had reached five steps in this time.

Obviously, you wouldn't expect Charlie to attempt the 130 meter walk I was doing, just as you wouldn't expect me to be able to jog that distance, I simply couldn't. Yet many people with ME/CFS have in effect done or been supervised to do something just as ridiculous for their circumstance, suffering weeks of PEM as a result. Hence, they've been put off any exercise by this i.e., **being unaware of their body's new level of limitation that ME/CFS has imposed.** This, now we understand ME/CFS better, can be avoided as you'll learn in coming chapters.

Mitochondrial Crash?

My time in rehabilitation got me reflecting on 24 years before. On July 17, 1996 when 'the plug was pulled' and my ME/CFS began - I felt deep sudden onset exhaustion, and I knew I was in serious trouble straight away. So, what happened? It felt like, perhaps, my body systems and mitochondria in particular, had finally tipped over an abyss; a severe (autoimmune induced?) inner crash much less visible yet just as

CHAPTER 11 THE ART OF MICRO-REHAB

impactful as Charlie's less hidden motor vehicle crash!

Perhaps these now 'shocked' mitochondria would require, like Charlie, a very gentle rehabilitation program to allow them and other systems to 'come back online,' a real possibility given our new understanding of epigenetics and neuroplasticity. Depending upon the severity of your illness, this process may need to be done over many months or years in baby-steps, much like Charlie.

I'd suggest progress is best judged long-term by returning function rather than the number of meters you can walk, although they often correlate. Hence, the focus of any exercise involved would be as an aid to function and have to be very carefully individualized.

For example, in 2004, after barely being able to walk 20 meters and needing to rest after this 20 meter effort, I was able to walk 2km after a year of ME/CFS paced rehab. To my joy, I found many other aspects of my ability to function, like stamina for standing, writing, reading, going out socializing etc. all had improved, a positive side-effect if you like.

Though I enjoyed sport and was very fit at different stages of my life, I was not a professional sportsman, so rather than continue to 'Grade up' my level of exercise I chose not to. Instead, I was happy to maintain the new level I'd achieved, walking 2 km every second day, with core muscle (Pilates) and light weights strengthening on other days. All up, I found around 30-45 minutes per day and one day off formal exercise per week was all I then needed to maintain better health and a better life. A price I was more than willing to pay.

Mitochondrial Repair?

Exactly how the right amount of exercise benefits ME/CFS is debated. We know in healthy people moderate exercise (where you get to the huff and puff stage but can still conduct a conversation) can result in improvements in blood flow, cognitive function, mood and immune function.[10] We also know that exercise in the right dose can improve mitochondrial (the cell's energy 'battery') function and even increases the number of mitochondria produced within each cell.[11]

As I have referred to in *A Doctor's Journey Back to Health*, rather than broken, as happens in forms of rare, severe genetic mitochondrial diseases that result in early death, what we have with ME/CFS is 'dysfunctional' mitochondria.[12] Dysfunctional mitochondria are still functioning but at a lower level of energy production. If we had more mitochondria within each cell, even if they were not functioning at their best, one would think it could only help one's overall energy production. So, this combined with improving mitochondrial efficiency via epigenetic phenomena may be a mechanism of improvement. We just don't know yet how this works; more research will be required.

Some have argued that the levels of exercise achieved by ME/CFS participants in an exercise program are not of a high enough intensity to cause such a benefit.[13] My experience and that of my patients suggests otherwise i.e., that any carefully paced increase in movement feels beneficial, and in time, there is a notable turning point, a physiological fitness and strength threshold if you like, which when reached, tips one back into a healthier more energetic state.

I'm not sure what happens biochemically, but I am sure about how it felt. It was as if the plug, after nine years on the outer, went back into the socket and the cell door of my low energy prison was opened, maybe not completely, but significantly.

I suspect future research will discover that while mitochondrial function may not return to 'normal' aerobic levels of function with gentle paced Micro-Rehab, in most people with ME/CFS, it can improve.

CHAPTER 11 THE ART OF MICRO-REHAB

How to Safely Introduce Exercise for people with ME/CFS

On the final day of the International ME/CFS Symposium on the Biomedical Basis of ME/CFS my wife, Tori, and I attended in March 2019,[14] I put this question to the expert clinical CFS panel, my question was as follows. "In my own clinical work with people with ME/CFS I'd found many had become so afraid of post exertional malaise (PEM) that they became afraid to move much at all. How do you approach this issue?" The four panelists were Dr Don Lewis, Dr Mark Donahoe, Dr Nicole Phillips and Dr Bruce Wauchope. They all agreed that they encouraged their patients to move as soon as they felt able to do so. The devil of course is in the detail of how to help people to do this without them freaking out, as I admit I initially did. When PEM strikes, you see, you don't know how long it's going to last for, so naturally you are going to need some very specific reassurance to overcome your fear of overdoing it or doing any exercise at all.

Fortunately, leading US ME/CFS physician's Dr Daniel Paterson and Dr Nancy Klimas together with exercise physiologists, including Connie Sol, have developed an approach for introducing exercise to people with ME/CFS that is safe, and are sharing this on a video.[15] The approach affirms what I discovered through my own experience and that of teaching my patients. Others have written about their own success with similar approaches.[16,17] Klimas's US team uses specialized equipment and expensive testing, including VO2 Max, not readily available to most people with ME/CFS, to guide their patient's rehab. Klimas now advises if done with care, exercise can be introduced without the expensive equipment.[18]

https://me-cfscommunity.com/

In the next chapter we'll look at how you can safely approach this without needing to use the VO2 Max testing used by Dr Klimas and her team. A heart rate monitor, a stationary (or reclining) exercise bike or foot cycle and the Borg RPE SCALE (see Ch 12) is all you'll need. Nonetheless, the video produced by Dr Klimas and Connie Sol which takes you through their approach with real ME/CFS patients (online purchase price $9.99US) is definitely worth a look. If you do this, I suggest you watch (but don't try out at this stage the exercise routine in it) the second half first, commencing at the 16-minute mark with Dan Moricoli's presentation, then returning to the beginning.[19]

Caution – we're all individuals

The one caution I'd give is not to copy any of the exercises shown in this or similar videos until you are properly assessed. You may be unaware of how much deconditioning you may have from months or years of inactivity. I was, and regrettably did not start by strengthening my core muscles first with Pilates-type exercises. Consequently, I ruptured two discs in my lower back. It delayed my life restoration by six months, and I learnt a valuable lesson but let me take that one for you!

If you can access and afford Dr Klimas's approach with practitioners experienced with ME/CFS and well calibrated razzle dazzle equipment, then by all means go for it. I have incorporated aspects of Dr Klimas's approach along with the approach I used successfully with my patients and will share my suggestions in full in Chapters 13-15.

Let's complete this chapter with a story that explores what a Micro-Rehab approach meant practically to a bedbound Samantha Miller, a London resident. First published in Jo Marchant's book, *Cure*,[20] I picked up Samantha's story from the Guardian.[21]

Samantha's Story

Samantha Miller, a 46-year old high school teacher and artist, developed a severe version of ME/CFS following several viral illnesses, a botched surgery and a high stress work environment, in which she

CHAPTER 11 THE ART OF MICRO-REHAB

felt trapped. Her recovery from ME/CFS was reported in London's Guardian newspaper in 2016.

To give you a sense of where Samantha was at before introducing a Rehab aspect into her management strategy, she described her experience with ME/CFS as feeling like she was being 'buried alive.' "I was exhausted, with terrible joint pains. It was like having the flu all the time with no certainty of recovery. I couldn't do anything. I was trapped."

When her father said, "This is boring. I think you should get better," Samantha was so hurt and fed up, she asked her partner and her sister to help her to kill herself. They eventually agreed, but only if she gave the paced rehab program at St Bartholomew's Hospital in London they'd recently discovered, a proper try for six months first. Samantha agreed.

- Samantha's first exercise goal was simply to turn over in bed once an hour. Every few days, she increased her activity slightly until she was able to sit up for five minutes at a time. When she was able, she kept an activity diary and as the months progressed, she was able to do more and see some progress. When she was finally out of bed, she got to the point where she might try cooking a meal, but the task would need to be split into small parts. Chop the onions. Go and lie down. Chop the carrots. Go and lie down etc. Each of these steps forward was the result of months of careful pacing and persistence.
- As a creative person, she found the total lack of spontaneity hard to accept. But the perfectionism that she feels contributed to her condition, helped her to persist.
- As she progressed, she recalls setting herself goals such as "walk to the next house and back." Then "walk two houses and back." Two weeks later she'd "walk for three houses and back." But jumping ahead and walking five houses and back might have put her in bed for three

weeks. She had to stick to the regime, doing no more and no less than the prescribed activity level, **no matter how good she was feeling.**

- If she pushed herself too hard, she would crash. "It takes incredible discipline," she says. "One slip-up and you (feel like) you are back to square one." If she broke the rules and tried to do too much, she would start to feel her body go. "I'd feel hot from the feet up, almost like I was being poisoned. Then I'd be ruined for weeks."

> **Note**: The mindful rest aspect of the rest activity dance you will learn soon can reduce setbacks and shorten restoration time if slip-ups do happen. It will be your secret weapon!

It took Samantha five years of grim determination, but she finally clawed her way out of the fatigue and pain and back into a normal life. She now works part-time, rides her bike and continues her passion as an artist.

The full Guardian article can be accessed at –

https://www.theguardian.com/society/2016/feb/15/it-was-like-being-buried-alive-victim-of-chronic-fatigue-syndrome

Chapter 11
Key Points

Micro-Rehab

- ✓ In ME/CFS overexertion worsens the condition whilst the right amount of activity can improve it.
- ✓ Hormesis is a concept of appropriate challenge to the whole person builds capacity.
- ✓ The focus of any carefully paced increase in movement is to aid function and has to be very carefully individualized. In this way it can be performed safely.
- ✓ Evidence suggests Micro-Rehab can rehabilitate dysfunctional mitochondria and improve symptoms.

Chapter 12

PREPARATION FOR EXERCISE

"By failing to prepare, you are preparing to fail."
BENJAMIN FRANKLIN

Take your time. Given the number of years this dreadful disease can take out of your life, a few weeks or a month devoted to getting yourself set up with the right supports, journal -including an activity log (see example below), equipment and a plan that feels safe and doable is truly worth it.

If it doesn't feel right or doable or just the word exercise gives you the 'willies' then try the relaxation exercises in the next chapter and/or the Defuse the Loop strategies in Chapter 15. Failing that you may need to dig a little deeper to see what is feeding this anxiety/fear, address it with your support crew (exercise physiologist/physio/GP, counsellor etc.) and come up with something, no matter how small, that does feel doable.

The first step is often the most challenging. But all you really need to do is something you can cope with and build from there. For example, supine exercising, that is exercising whilst lying on your back is the best place to start if you are either bedbound or have POTS or NMH leading to low blood pressure. Several of my POTS patients found Clinical Pilates on a Pilates Reformer under physiotherapy supervision was their exercise of choice at least to begin with.

The confidence you will gain from any small beginning will be extraordinary.

Helpful Equipment
- Biofeedback: A continuous Heat Rate Monitor, that can be strapped around your chest and signals a watch (or other mobile device) in real time. As you need to access this information during exercise, a chest strap and watch were my preference. However, there are a variety of clips on an earlobe or finger that can also be used.
- A pedometer may also be useful.
- Resistance bands (stretchy exercise bands available in sports shops, Kmart and online. Start with the yellow one). You can even use these in bed if required.
- Overhanging bed-pole may be helpful if you are bed bound. You can use it as a mobility aid and to attach resistance bands too for strengthening exercises. A Physio or Occupational Therapist (OT) may need to set it up.
- Timer Apps can be useful if you want to ensure you don't overdo it.
- Yoga mat to stretch, rest or do Yoga poses upon. (Clinical Pilates, individualized Yoga and TaiChi were helpful for some of my patients.)
- Foot Cycle (Mini Exercise bike in Kmart), Stationary or reclining exercise bike. Foot cycles are inexpensive around $30.00AUS. (If you have POTS or NMH a reclining exercise bike or rowing machine may be preferable).

Rating of Perceived Exertion (RPE)

Familiarize yourself with the Rating of Perceived Exertion (Borg RPE) scale below.[1]

If your level of effort reaches 7 or more then if possible, to avoid PEM, stop and rest. As I explained in my book *A Doctor's Journey Back to*

Health Ch 11, because of problems with the autonomic nervous system in ME/CFS, such as chronotropic intolerance (CI) where the heart rate rises sluggishly, a heart rate monitor is less reliable for self-monitoring than your RPE score, at least initially. Remember we are talking about your RPE or current effort level NOW. Not what you were able to do prior to developing ME/CFS.

Until your heart rate synchronizes with your RPE it's best avoided as a complete guide to your rehabilitation. If you do exceed an RPE of 7, then aim to minimize this to no more than 90 seconds and follow this with a rest of at least double this amount of time, as I will teach you in the next chapter.

1-2	No effort at all
2-3	minimal effort
3-4	Extremely light effort
4-5	Very Light (e.g., walking slowly at your own pace)
5-6	Light
6-7	Somewhat hard. You start to huff & puff but can still conduct a conversation if needs be. (You feel OK to continue, YET – this is where I suggest you STOP initially (i.e., during the first 3 months) and mindfully rest, so you can bank the benefit and build your energy account/resilience.)
7-8	Hard
8-9	Very Hard
10	Maximal exertion

Table 1 Rating of Perceived Exertion (RPE)[1]

Resting Morning Heart Rate

In keeping an activity log (see below) for at least a week prior to introducing anything new, it will be useful to record your resting morning heart rate (RMHR). This is how you do it: - For one week after waking, before rising, drinking/eating or taking any medication, attach your heart rate monitor and lay flat on your back for 10 minutes, with a pillow under your head. Record the lowest heart rate level reached. This will give you an accurate reading of your resting morning heart rate (RMHR).

Over the week you will generally find the lowest HR that your heart reaches at rest. Mine was unusually low at 42 beats per minute (bpm). [Note: A HR Monitor is 10 to 15% more accurate than simply taking your own pulse.]

If during your paced rehab program, you find this resting morning heart rate is 8% or more above the usual RMHR it usually indicates your body is battling on some level (e.g., a cold or previous over-exertion). For example, if mine was 46 bpm this would be 10% higher than my usual RMHR of 42.

In this situation it is best either to not exercise that day or reduce your routine by half, just so you keep things moving gently, as I would tend to do.

For this reason, I suggest initially that you wear a continuous heart rate monitor and keep an activity log (as set out below) for a week before introducing any exercise sessions.

I would also suggest you find yourself an appropriately ME/CFS-experienced exercise physiologist or physiotherapist. If this ME/CFS expertise is not available where you are, or too difficult to access, you could ask your treating practitioner if they are willing to learn. If so, you may wish to share this book (or direct them to the relevant exercise bits i.e., Chapters 8 to 14).

CHAPTER 12 PREPARATION FOR EXERCISE

Mobility Aid

If you do use an indoor stationary exercise bike or foot-cycle I suggest you first use it like a mobility aid. By mobility aid, I do not mean for walking, I mean you roll your legs cycling gently for no more than 10 seconds at least twice a day. This will at least get your leg joints and blood flow moving a little. But what I want you to achieve most of all is familiarity with what I hope will become your new best healing friend(s). After these 10 second mobility leg rolls, practice resting briefly, taking several slow deep breaths for at least half a minute.

If you are bedbound and have a willing helper, a foot cycle can be positioned on your bed and stabilized by your helper (minding their fingers) whilst you cycle with your legs. This is the most inexpensive way of creating a reclining bicycle and you can advance to sitting on the edge of your bed or a chair and foot cycling from there when you're able.

A big advantage of this equipment is it allows you to standardize your efforts indoors with windows open to allow airflow, regardless of the weather outside. On cold rainy days, by the time I'd put my gear on I was too tired to walk, not that I want to put you off walking. It's just your improvement will be steadier if you also have a familiar indoor option on bad weather days.

Activity Log

Begin with what you are doing right now and keep an Activity Log (see below) for one week whilst wearing a heart rate monitor. Do not add any extra activities for this initial 7 day recording period. On waking each morning record your resting morning heart rate (RMHR), as described above. Then during or immediately after each main activity, record your peak Rating of Perceived Exertion (RPE) and heart rate (HR). In this way you will be seeing how these two measures relate to each other so you can become more self-aware of your body signals and what they mean.

Leading ME/CFS researchers now suggest that if you can keep your heart rate below 60% (some say 65%) of the maximum level recommended for a healthy individual, and not exceed 90 seconds at this level of HR at one-time, you will not trigger PEM. How good is that piece of info![2]

HR Max Calculation

Your 60% maximum recommended HR is calculated by subtracting your age from 220 and multiplying this by 0.60 (ie 60%). For example, in 2004 when I began a similar program to what I'm presenting here, I was 43 years old. Hence the calculation was 220-43 = 177 x 0.60 = 106.

In 2004 I was unaware of this 60% suggestion. Yet using the RPE as a guide rather than heart rate (recall I had Chronotropic Intolerance) I was able to slowly add 15 seconds of stationary bike cycling every two to four weeks to my second daily (initially just 30 second) cycling routine. In time when my routine reached around 3 minutes of cycling, my heart rate started to increase more naturally in tune with the RPE. It was then I recognized that I needed to keep my heart rate below 110 to be safe from triggering an episode of PEM. In noting your heart rate and RPE during your daily activities you will also get a sense of which activities are the most taxing and may need to be paced differently e.g., broken up with a brief rest or different easier activity.

For example, if you find walking up a flight of stairs raises your HR above your 60% ceiling, then you could try walking up the stairs more slowly or resting half-way up and see which strategies keep the HR below this ceiling whilst still achieving the task of getting to the top of the stairs.

Below is an example of my activity log, prior to introducing exercise.

Day	Night sleep Hrs	RMHR	MAIN ACTIVITIES & EVENTS	Cycle Indoor	Rating of Perceived Exertion (RPE) 1-10	Peak HR	Symptoms	Severity (0 - 10)
MON	7	52	Shower hair wash		7	84	Fatigue	8
TUES	8	56	5 mins gardening weeding		8	112	Headache	6
WEDS	5	62	5 mins stressful phone call Constipation		8	106	PEM fatigue muscle pain, brain fog	9
THURS	10	60	Food prep		5-6	80	PEM	9
FRID	12	54	Rest		4	66	PEM	9
SAT	12	52	Rest		5	58		7
SUN	10	52	Shower		4	72		5
MON	8	52		Cycle 30 secs	6	56	Muscle soreness	6
TUES	7	54	LIGHT WTS 5 min		4	58	soreness	5

Muscle Pain

A warning, because your muscles will have reduced in size during months of debility there may be an increase in muscle soreness/achiness when beginning to move more. This is usually short-lived and improves with rest after a couple of days. There can also be some Delayed Onset Muscle Soreness (DOMS), which can be a normal response to this unfamiliar increase in movement. It is easy to fear that this is the beginning of a crash i.e., Post-Exertional Malaise, a fear we will learn how to defuse in Chapters 13 and 15. Hence, it is important to learn to differentiate between the two; PEM being more flu-like aching with brain fog, while DOMS is typically experienced after a delay of 24 to 48 hours after exercise as muscle soreness, weakness and stiffness which can last 3 to 7 days.[3,4]

The DOMS-type of soreness is acceptable. When you have pain

that is a feeling of soreness or achiness, it's usually the result of mild inflammation, or microtears in your muscles or tendons. This is normal. The muscle repairs these tears when you're resting, and this helps muscles grow in size and strength. This microtrauma may sound harmful, but it is your body's natural response when your muscles experience work.[5]

Even though we've learnt in Chapter 10 and 12 in my previous book (*A Doctor's Journey Back to Health*) that people with ME/CFS have low grade inflammation and less production of heat shock protein (which assists in muscle repair and growth), this does not mean it needs to be avoided altogether.[6] It is in fact a good example of hormesis; appropriate challenge builds resilience, as despite this limitation, the muscles of people with ME/CFS can and do improve strength and resilience, they just need to build more slowly.

The take home message is that a certain low level of soreness is acceptable, physical activity may even ease the achiness, but you should not push through pain while exercising. Overall, most people I saw who stayed within their limits were surprised how their headaches and muscle pain generally improved. We now know that whilst overexertion causes pain in ME/CFS by the release of inflammatory cytokines, so too not moving much causes the release of similar inflammatory cytokines also leading to pain.[7] We were meant to move, with ME/CFS, it's just a question of how much.

Alastair Lynch's Story

Let's conclude this chapter with the uplifting story of well-known Australian Rules Football champion Alastair Lynch. His brush with ME/CFS almost ended his flourishing career. His book, *Taking Nothing for Granted – a Sportsman's fight with Chronic Fatigue*[8] inspired me not to give up and gave me some of the clues that would help me to restore

CHAPTER 12 PREPARATION FOR EXERCISE

much of my life and eventually lead me to developing the approach I'm teaching you in this book.

> In September 1994 Alastair Lynch was 25 years of age with a bright future beckoning. A big, strapping man at the top of his game, he was considered amongst the best Australian Rules footballers in the country. He had just relocated his family from Melbourne to Brisbane where he had joined the Brisbane Lions Football Club. A number of other major stressors in his life (a home burglary, car accident and a death in the family) culminated in him contracting a nasty viral illness, which he could not seem to shake. It left him sleeping 18 hours a day and experiencing the full gamut of ME/CFS symptoms.
>
> Over the ensuing months he consulted more than 40 practitioners, including many medical specialists. Eventually a diagnosis of CFS was made. As his debility dragged on, he was desperate for answers. He even flew to the US to consult with a CFS specialist. In his frank and readable book, he outlines his story, including the following remarks about his rehabilitation:
>
> "Dr Whiting and the football club's medical and conditioning team and I had together formulated an exercise program which allowed me to train without suffering the most severe effects of CFS. The program started with very light weights and minimal exercise. I would lift 30–40 per cent of my normal capacity and slowly graduate from short walks to slow jogs. There's a fine line, which only the patient can judge. My program was to do a little but not make myself tired, and make sure I gave myself plenty of rest. I started off lifting 20kg on a bench press and walking 200 metres.
>
> I believed then and still believe that exercise is most important. But it's difficult to identify exactly how much exercise is optimal.

> In my experience, CFS sufferers need to stimulate their bodies (Note: Alastair also found ice baths helpful - for my suggestions re cold showers see the end of this chapter). As much as they might feel like spending all day in bed when CFS is at its peak, it doesn't do any good. They've got to do a little something, and gradually build it up. Even if it's only walking to the letterbox or to the local shops if they are close by. Patients need to listen to their body: it provides the best guide to the middle ground between enough exercise and too much. Err on the cautious side, I'd say, because it's easy to overdo it. And be patient. It's always going to take time."

Alastair recovered enough from CFS to return to playing professional football 12 months later. His capacities were limited compared to what he was able to do prior to developing CFS. He had an individualized training regime that differed from his teammates and on match days was confined to playing on the forward line, where he could rest frequently between bursts of activity. The club also discovered there was no point flying him from Brisbane to Perth to play because two five-hour plus flights crashed his energy levels for the following week. In contrast two-hour flights for matches in Melbourne were tolerated.

- With careful management he was able to make a significant contribution to the team, a team considered one of the best in the history of AFL football. By the time he retired in 2004, he had been the leading goal scorer in three premiership games. Note: In 2018 SBS television in Australia included Alastair on a panel discussing CFS, see link - https://www.sbs.com.au/ondemand/video/1334946883764/insight-chronic-fatigue-syndrome

In his book, Alastair points out he is not the only professional sportsperson to experience CFS. Other well-known Australians include,

CHAPTER 12 PREPARATION FOR EXERCISE

seven-time world surfing champion Layne Beachley, Olympic kayak gold medalist Clint Robinson, marathon swimmer Shelley Taylor-Smith, former Test cricketers Simon Katich and Matthew Nicholson, triathlete Craig Walton, swimmers Duncan Armstrong and Linley Frame, and ex-swimmer turned television personality Johanna Griggs.

It is curious to me that most of the stories I've read or heard of involving professional sports people finds them able to recover from CFS, partially and rarely fully, within the relatively short time of 1 to 2 years. It makes me wonder what the factors are that allow them to do so? I suspect the support they receive and their familiarity with exercise and ability to commit to a disciplined, Micro-Rehab program, learning how to not over train i.e., push themselves, is likely to be among the most important reasons.

Rosamund Valling, an experienced New Zealand-based GP and author with over 40 years-experience in treating people with ME/CFS, emphasizes the opposite fact. She found athletes often would struggle to learn how to pace and in continuing to push they'd typically go downhill.[8] Maybe it's only the ones, like Alastair, who learn the discipline of a Micro-Rehab type approach who end up writing books about their success!!

As Alastair wisely emphasized, *"Patients need to listen to their body: it provides the best guide to the middle ground between enough exercise and too much. Err on the cautious side, I'd say, because it's easy to overdo it. And be patient. It's always going to take time."*[10]

Note: As mentioned earlier, Alastair also found **ice baths** to be helpful, particularly with brain fog. This might be OK for larger bodied people and you might build towards this, but what I'd suggest is:

Try **ending your showers cooler** by slowly turning down the hot water as you increase the cold, all the while breathing gently into your belly. Once again, the concept of **hormesis** applies here - Appropriate challenge builds strength. If you feel like upping the antie (maybe on a warmer day to begin with) keep the cold water running and turn off the hot water completely, keep focusing on your breathing, slowly into your belly– this gets easier with practice – it helps me as the water gets colder to imagine I'm being cleansed in a refreshing ocean.

Aim to stay under the cold shower for just a few seconds to start with, building up to seven slow belly breaths (approx. 30 seconds.). This can clear brain fog, stimulate a rebalance of your immune system and may have other health benefits.[11]

Think of the warm shower being for your body and cold shower for your brain. Wrap yourself in a warm towel when finished.

Chapter 12
Key Points

- ✓ In most endeavors in life preparation is the key to success.
- ✓ I suggest indoor equipment at home (rented if needs be) so that you can exercise even if the weather outside is not conducive.
- ✓ At a minimum a yoga mat, heart rate (HR) monitor and foot cycle.
- ✓ Familiarize yourself with the Rating of Perceived Exertion (RPE) scale. It will help to guide your activity keeping within 65% of your maximum capacity.
- ✓ Keep an Activity log similar to the one I've included for at least 7 days before adding any new movement, recording RPE and HR so that you can learn how the two align for you.
- ✓ To improve your situation as Alastair Lynch and Samantha Miller's (see previous chapter) examples

demonstrate, you will need to increase your level of activity safely. For most people, like Samantha and Alastair, you will need professional guidance with this (e.g., physio, exercise physiologist.)
- ✓ The key is to find your minimal activity level that you can safely do and build from there. For bedbound Samantha it was rolling over in bed once every hour. For Alastair it was slowly walking 200 metres, then resting.
- ✓ Some immediate or delayed onset muscle soreness (DOMS) is likely as muscles are being asked to do more. This is a good thing as it means your muscles are getting stronger. In time you will learn how to clearly distinguish this from the flu-like Post Exertional Malaise (PEM).
- ✓ Consider ending your shower cool to help brain fog. A warm shower for your body and a cool one for your mind.

Chapter 13
STOP! THE REST ACTIVITY DANCE

"Take rest: a field that has rested gives a bountiful crop."
OVID

Micro-Rehab is different to exercise in two very important ways. The first way I have already discussed at length and relates to staying strictly within your energy envelope and increasing your program sub-maximally according to perceived effort on the RPE scale and your heart rate (HR). The other essential ingredient of Micro-Rehab is **mindful rest**.

Rest is an equal partner in the dance. It may even be the first step. It is the secret ingredient to allowing your body to integrate and accommodate to the greater demand of moving more again. Hence, I call it the Rest/Activity Dance.

Beginning and completing an activity session with gentle stretching, mindful breathing and a deep relaxation or meditation can be profoundly beneficial. Don't underestimate the restoring powers of deep rest.

Tuning In

To introduce the idea of mindful rest let's firstly take a look at the Fight/Flight or Stress response. This response is activated when we find ourselves under threat or feeling awkward or out of our depth. It can also be triggered by fears and negative thoughts we may not even realize we are having (see Chapter 15). When we are embarking on a new rehabilitation program and demanding new movements and effort from our body in the grips of ME/CFS, it is not just a physical rehabilitation that we are undertaking. We are needing to relearn trust in our body. This means we also need to integrate the new messages from our body about what we can safely accomplish. We have had a multitude of negative experiences in the form of post-exertional malaise (PEM) that have told us that we are no longer in control of our bodily reactions.

Rehabilitation, no matter how carefully paced may be unfamiliar to us and we don't know how our body will respond. This is the inner battle. As we've discussed, most of us with the condition have had bad experiences with exercise when we have done too much and suffered in ways that are vastly disproportionate to the effects on a healthy person. Therefore, any mode of rehabilitation may feel potential risky, even if we are not immediately aware of it. If this is the case and your body and mind are tense, unable to find rest, then neither your RPE nor HR will be optimal as effective guides to gauging the safe amount of activity. In this situation I suggest you look at the rest of this chapter, along with the Defuse the Loop (Chapter 15) before moving to Chapter 14.

The Stress Response

In any stressful situation, nerves fire impulses and chemicals, and hormones are released that tighten muscles, increase our heart rate and blood pressure and cause rapid shallow breathing. This can be useful if we need to fight or take evasive action, like jumping out of the way of a bus. But when it is switched on by a chronic and relentless illness like ME/CFS, where brainstem inflammation appears to be driving the Autonomic Nervous System (ANS) towards a sympathetic overdrive, stress is a constant presence in our lives rather than a healthy intermittent state of heightened alertness.

CHAPTER 13 STOP! THE REST ACTIVITY DANCE

As discussed in my previous book, in people prone to ME/CFS there appears to be a hypometabolic or hibernation-like state triggered by serious threats be they infective, physical or psychological in people with ME/CFS. This appears to be linked to the brainstem and can lead to the distinctive pattern of symptoms seen in ME/CFS.

In addition to all of this, unchecked, in time, stress develops its own momentum, and this can lead to chronic stress. In this situation we can become so used to its presence, that we live life in its shadow. It combines and can perpetuate our ME/CFS symptoms. It exacerbates the problems with our health and happiness, and further disturbs our concentration. ME/CFS can already impact on our relationships, and internal or external stress can multiply it. **If we can reduce this anxiousness, then our energies can be focused on managing the main game**.

Fortunately, there is an antidote parasympathetic response that we can all learn to invoke at will, the Relaxation Response (RR), and it is this response that is our dance partner in Micro-Rehab.

The Relaxation Response

In the late 1960's Harvard University cardiologist, Dr Herbert Benson, became interested in researching the effects of Eastern meditation techniques arriving in the U.S at the time. He even took his equipment to the east to study meditating monks. In time he researched a variety of meditation and relaxation techniques and he identified a bodily response that they all had in common. He called this response the relaxation response and published a book with this title in 1975.[1] During the relaxation response, heart and breathing rates slow, blood pressure lowers, muscles relax, and the body receives a deeper restorative rest than at any time during sleep. We are happily relaxed while at the same time clearly awake.

Subsequent research has shown that the relaxation response can be switched on in a variety of ways. Deep breathing, meditation, progressive muscle relaxation, visualization, repetitive prayer, tai chi, yoga, knitting the list goes on. Personal preference plays a part. For instance, knitting would not be my first choice for switching off, while for others it is their 'meditation' of choice.

Importantly, all these activities require our active participation and give our minds something to focus upon. In other words, paradoxically, while the stress response is often triggered without us knowing, the relaxation response requires our conscious efforts, hence I call it mindful rest. Furthermore, Dr Benson's research found that if someone practiced a focused relaxation technique for as little as 10 minutes a day, after just one month their quality of life and ability to cope with stress had all improved.

Learning how to invoke this response with techniques that can be used anywhere and anytime is a wonderful life skill. The Rest/Activity dance means that when you complete a physical movement or activity in your Micro-Rehab program it is not finished until you have also completed a period of mindful rest.

It is very beneficial to become aware of how much rest your body requires to feel restored from an amount of effort. This period of mindful rest helps you to do this. It reinforces the relaxation response, helps the deconditioned muscles to recover, helps your heart to recover fitness and is invaluable in helping you to discern how long your body requires to recover from activity generally. If it is taking **more than 30 minutes** of mindful rest to feel the activity is integrated (bodily restored), it usually means you've done too much physical activity. Becoming familiar with this feeling of physical recovery after exertion will assist in building mind-body trust.

Rest also helps you to hear some of the inner fearful self-talk that may be going on in your mind and helps you to build internal awareness (we will focus more on this in Chapter 15).

I will give you instructions here and in the Appendices of this book for all the techniques I used with my patients. Some of my techniques are literally one breaths duration. Some of them are longer. You do not have to spend hours meditating to achieve the relaxation response, in fact it is often more beneficial to start with a very brief technique.

There are also innumerable relaxation, mindfulness and meditation sites online. (E.g., www.smilingmind.com.au and www.headspace.org.au)

Alternatively, you can listen to and follow along with the meditations and relaxations I am sharing with you here (See Appendices 5 & 6) and on my Download, Restoring Balance, that can be found on my website at www.drstevensommer.com.

Brain Science & Benefits

Neuroscientists now inform us that the brain keeps forming new connections throughout our lives. We can think of our brains as growing new branches like a tree in response to the inputs we give to it. As I've mentioned before this is called **neuroplasticity** and it explains why we can get better at something the more we practice it, at any age. It also means that if the stress response is being activated regularly, more pathways quite literally form in our brains to make this response happen more easily. Fortunately, regularly triggering the relaxation response (RR) leads the stress pathways to lose their pre-eminent position. In time, these stress connections will resemble slow overgrown tracks while the relaxation pathways will form paved freeways. In other words, if you practice letting go and relaxing, you will get better at it. Even if some find this easier to learn than others, like writing, we can all do it.

There are many benefits of regularly switching on the RR. The most obvious is reducing anxiety, improving mood and sleep and simply allowing us to feel more joy in our lives, or at least reminding us to appreciate what we can do rather than what we can't yet do.

When we integrate the relaxation response in our Micro-Rehab program, we gain a double benefit of helping our physical bodies to integrate the new activity and our minds to settle and trust the process. As we take these short time outs from our daily struggle with our illness, we can also find that our ability to tune into our intuition improves. This helps us to solve problems, be more creative and make better decisions. This has positive implications in terms of helping us take up the healthier habits that can help us to manage ME/CFS, rather than it manage us. I have also seen it benefit people dealing with addictions, like smoking or alcohol.

Other health benefits are numerous. Blood pressure can improve, our immune system can regulate itself better, so we have fewer crash days, while sugar metabolism also benefits, thus helping diabetics and those with hypoglycemia. Learning to relax has been an important part of Cardiac Rehabilitation too for some years now.[2]

It is also worth noting that anxiety and tension not only contribute to fatigue but can also turn up the volume on pain. As muscle tension and anxiety decrease, headaches (including migraine) and chronic pain diminish. This is good news for those whose illness includes chronic pain.

Resetting your stress thermostat

We all have a stress thermostat, a barometer if you like, which determines how easily or not we become stressed. It is located in the brainstem and when it is raised high as it often is in ME/CFS, we can become anxious very easily, when it is set low, we are more resistant to stress. Our genetics, upbringing, brainstem inflammation, illnesses and life traumas can all affect our thermostat. Fortunately, regardless of where it sits today, the choices you make now and from now on can influence it as well.

The basis of the Rest/Activity dance is to learn to **punctuate** our Micro-Rehab active sessions with brief techniques that induce the RR. 'Commas' are brief pauses that can take as little as thirty seconds, while 'Full Stops' require a minimum of five minutes of mindful rest. When this is combined with the techniques I will share with you in Chapter 15, Defuse the Loop, it can help to improve your ME/CFS symptoms as chronic tension is released.

The First Comma

Two slow breaths can be taken at any time in your day, helping you to rebalance. I refer to this as a pause or comma. The breath is the most direct method for activating the relaxation response and it takes only a couple of minutes to tune into and learn this technique.

If you are not already lying down, then lay down on your back on a comfortable surface with your head supported on a pillow. If your ME/CFS is severe, particularly if you are bed bound, then this is the safest and most effective strategy in this book with which to start your Micro-Rehab program. So, let's continue.

I want you to place one of your hands on your chest, over your heart area and place your other hand on your lower belly, prop your elbow up with a pillow if necessary. And just continue to breathe normally. There is no need to try to breathe more deeply in this exercise. Let the breath flow in and out as it normally does, it might take a few breaths for it to resume what feels like normal to you.

I want you to focus your attention on your hands. Notice the movement of your hands as they move with your breathing. Pay attention to the sensation on the surface of your palms on your skin or your clothing. Notice if one hand is moving more than the other. Allow yourself time to examine this, this will tell you where your breath is flowing to. Is it more pronounced under the hand on your chest or is it more noticeable under the hand on your belly? For some people it might feel the same under both hands. There is no right way, it's just a matter of noticing what your body is doing right now.

Once you feel like you have a good idea of what you are feeling with your hands and how much they are moving with your breathing, I want you, without tipping your head back, to look upwards with your eyes. Allow your eyes to look up comfortably, without straining, towards the top of your head. Then, maintaining your upward gaze, notice your hands again. Is there any change in how the breath is moving under your hands? Is it more noticeable under one hand than the other? Has it changed hands or changed volume, has it changed in rate or has it remained the same? Simply notice for three breaths then lower your eyes again. Take a moment to notice how you feel having completed the exercise.

This is your first comma in the Rest/Activity dance. Once you have practiced it several times lying down and become familiar with it, it can be done seated or in any position you can safely look up with your eyes towards the top of your head. It can be done standing still but remember not to tip your head back, just look upwards with your eyes. Tipping your head back can cause dizziness and loss of balance. Once you can feel where your breath is going, try without your hands in position. The secret is to look up and notice what happens to your breathing. If this technique feels good to you, try introducing it regularly into your day. For example, before and after each meal or whenever you're sitting on the loo. It is the beginning of creating a relaxation response (RR) highway in your brain, one that in time, will supersede the stress response relegating it to a back road.

TABLE 1 A Comma in your Day

**Chapter 13
Key Points**

- ✓ The relaxation response (RR) was first described in the 1970's by US cardiologist Herbert Benson and is an antidote to the stress response.
- ✓ Learning how to evoke this regularly during the day can reduce anxiety, pain and stress.
- ✓ It is your secret weapon in becoming more active. Incorporating it into the Rest/Activity Dance as an equal partner so that the dance is only complete after you invoke this RR, will help to ensure the activity is integrated. Ultimately this will help you to build mind-body trust again, listening to and responding to your body's needs.
- ✓ With regular practice, neuroplasticity will encourage the brain pathways that give you the ability to mindfully rest rather than stress to predominate. This can be a great reassurance and comfort during your ME/CFS journey and helps you to build self-awareness and intuition so that making better choices becomes easier.

Chapter 14

GO... GENTLY! THE REST/ACTIVITY DANCE

"Be not afraid of growing slowly..."
CHINESE PROVERB

"Once I saw the importance of exercise and started to exercise regularly. I noticed many benefits, such as decreased fatigue during the day and better sleep at night. Now I wish that I had introduced exercise into my recovery regime two or three years earlier."
JOHANNES, ME/CFS BLOG[1]

Now that we have learnt how to stop, it's time to learn how to go... gently!

Some years back I attended a presentation by Professor Stephen Chang, a professor of Traditional Chinese Medicine based in Singapore. There was one thing he suggested that flipped my thinking about how we in the West approach physical activity. Professor Chang suggested something outrageous, "there should be an Olympic event where the winner is the **slowest** person over 100 metres."

Reflect on that for a second. Not riveting entertainment perhaps, but masterful, nonetheless.

It is in the spirit of this flip in looking at this new 'Olympic event' that I want you to approach this Chapter. For when it comes to Micro-Rehab, we are moving ever so slightly further on from pacing alone. Why bother? When we learn how Micro-Rehab can be done without inducing post exertional malaise (PEM), as my patients and others have discovered, then it allows us to not only develop more health and stamina, but critically to feel more of a sense of control over ME/CFS, rather than it over us.

After three months or so setback-free, you'll be the one calling the shots and your stamina and symptoms will noticeably improve.

Once again, the principle of hormesis applies here, appropriate challenge strengthens. So obviously, each person's starting point will be different.

Check in with your GP Before Commencing

Any exercise program needs to be individualized. People may have other issues that need to be considered and possibly treated before a rehabilitation program can be safely devised. For example, people may have asthma or low blood pressure or a post-Covid 19 illness with ongoing heart and lung damage and symptoms such as breathlessness. Once symptoms are adequately managed some appropriate rehabilitation should be possible for all.

Where to begin?

By now you may already have created an Activity Log and recorded some entries into it (see Chapter 12). If not, before adding any new activities, spend at least a week recording your log. Start with what you are doing right now and keep this Activity Log accessible (e.g., An app on your phone or on your iPad or a spreadsheet on the fridge) so you can add to it.

After each main activity, like after dressing, record your peak Rating of Perceived Exertion (RPE) and heart rate (HR). Recall from Chapter 12, in this way you will be seeing how these two measures relate to each other so you can become more self-aware of your body signals and what they mean.

CHAPTER 14 GO... GENTLY! THE REST/ACTIVITY DANCE

If Chronotropic Intolerance, a sluggish increase in HR in response to exercise, is a significant problem, as it was for me, then RPE (below 7 out of 10) will be a more reliable indicator than HR initially, although as I found, after 3 months or so, HR became useful too. If this is not an issue and HR correlates appropriately with RPE, aim to keep your heart rate at or below 60% of the maximum level recommended for a healthy individual of your age (i.e., 220 - your age x 60%).

If you are not sure which measure to rely upon (RPE or HR) keep recording both and if in doubt use the limit reached first (i.e., RPE 7 or HR 60% of Max). Once you negotiate this level of effort safely, then this is your starting point to build your program from.

For example, initially it might take 15 seconds or up to a minute of 'rolling' your legs on the foot cycle to reach your RPE of 7. At this point you go for another 15 seconds, then stop and lay down knees bent or flat, and rest. As I said before (see Chapter 12) as long as you keep the level of aerobic activity below 90-seconds duration you're unlikely to experience PEM, especially if you follow this activity immediately with mindful restful belly breathing. **Sub-maximal effort** is the key – always end feeling like you could do more and as with pacing, timetable to follow any activity with focused relaxation.

Let me further delineate what I mean by introducing more 'activity.'

Passive Activity – The most ill bedbound people with CFS who cannot move at all, may need a physiotherapist to passively move their joints through a range of motion. The physio could potentially teach carers or a physio aid to do this once or twice a day to begin with.

Maintenance Activity - What you're able to do right now without causing PEM. E.g., wriggling your fingers and toes, rolling over in bed, sitting up and feeding yourself, walking to the toilet and back (with or without assistance), walking to the letter box and back etc. This tolerated activity needs to continue on a daily basis.

Core muscle Strength and Stretching – This can be done every day. Learning to activate your core muscles is very helpful and can even be done whilst in bed. This skill can enable you to activate these core muscles during day to day activities and this can reduce pain and prevent injury to your back. Most physiotherapists can teach you this. Clinical Pilates using a piece of equipment known as a Pilates Reformer may also be helpful for those well enough to do this and as I've said, people with low blood pressure issues like NMH or POTS could consider this type of rehabilitation with a physio, as it can be done in a lying down position.

Resistance Bands, light weights, hydrotherapy. Depending on your preference and situation choose one of these to join with core muscle work. Start off timetabling this 2 to 3 x per week (never on consecutive days). Alternate with aerobic days.

Aerobic - Always limit this to every second day. This is the exercise ME/CFS groups advise their members to rightly be careful with. Walking, jogging, swimming and cycling are all considered aerobic activities, **anything that elevates your heart rate and/or makes you puff**.

The trick I found here, particularly with any aerobic forms of exercise, is that to begin with you start off feeling crappy then usually reach a point where you're feeling better and naturally want to continue. This is the point to **STOP**, sit or lie down and actively mindfully relax or meditate. Allow your body to integrate the effort. (See Chapter 13 and Appendices 5 & 6)

Sub-max Rehab

In doing sub-maximal rehabilitation in this way you sacrifice a little bit of short-term feeling good for the longer-term benefits of feeling consistently better. Remember, this is **Micro-Rehab as medicine.** We are talking about revitalizing confidence; muscle strength and tone; blood flow that assists brain fog; rehabbing the Autonomic Nervous System and the immune systems; and improving the body's ability to detoxify.[2,3]

Pacing your rehabilitation like this, you can learn to stop before you over do it. This gets easier to do as you identify the target level of effort which is your optimal point to reach and STOP at. For a certain level of activity you will find as you repeat the rehabilitation sessions at this level over weeks or months you will require less effort to do so, perhaps your RPE rating will drop from 7 to 5 out of 10 and/or HR from 60 to 50% max.

When this occurs during your second daily aerobic activity days, consistently for **at least** two weeks or more, you can gradually increase your activity level (by 15 seconds every 2 to 4 weeks) challenging yourself enough to reach a 6 to 7 RPE level of effort again. Repeat this gentle process each time it becomes easier i.e., the RPE drops below 6 and/or HR below 50% max), increasing the challenge 2 to 4 weekly. Even if this feels too easy, only increase the exercise time again after you have spent at least 2 weeks at this next level.

Educate your Therapist(s)

A **caution** here, most physiotherapists and exercise physiologists I and others with ME/CFS have consulted with did not understand the level of debility this illness causes. They would therefore suggest starting levels of exercise prescription way above what we as patients could safely do. Just as previously noted, medication and natural therapy dosages need to be much lower for people with ME/CFS than healthy people, so too starting exercise dosages.

Rehabilitation professionals often simply lacked the training to work with people this gently. For example, even strength work using yellow resistant bands would be prescribed as 10 repetitions followed by a minute's rest and another 10 reps.

I would suggest starting with two repetitions, a 30-60 second rest, then two more reps. Build up from 2 to 10 reps over at least two months. Once you have a congruent, safe starting point, then together with your therapist you should be able to devise a suitably individualized plan to follow and safely increase with.

Terrain Changing Magic

The magic of this is, while it may take months or years, as this process continues you will gradually and then sometimes with exponential leaps, increase your stamina, wellbeing and level of activity, expanding your energy envelope in ALL parts of your life. It seems that the mitochondria may be able to be rehabilitated after all. Nonetheless, recall Caitlin's cautionary tale (see Chapter 6) of burning her reserves all at once, and remember to continue to pace your day according to your energy envelope.

It would be fascinating to see some research on this observation. Could these increases in energy apply to all people with ME/CFS or just particular subtypes? Apart from comparing subtypes, I also now believe our research protocols in terms of assessing holistic 'terrain' treatments require a longer-term view of at least two to three years. Just as with the five-year follow up studies with MS (see Ch 2), analysis would need to include compliance with the holistic lifestyle changes, study and/or work capacity, standardized physical, quality of life and psychological measures as well as genomic comparisons.

Below in Table 1 is a review summary of the keys to Micro-Rehab.

Following this I'll share with you Katie's story, someone with whom I consulted who followed this approach with considerable success.

CHAPTER 14 GO... GENTLY! THE REST/ACTIVITY DANCE

- If possible, consult with an exercise physiologist or physiotherapist with expertise in ME/CFS rehabilitation to receive an individualized program. This individualized approach can encompass the range of severity and subgroups of people affected by ME/CFS, as it is guided by an accurate assessment of your symptoms and capabilities and built upon from there.
- Familiarize yourself with the RPE scale (Chapter 12) whilst doing your usual current routine.
- Purchase a continuous heart rate (HR) monitor to help guide your efforts.
- Log Activity for 7 days before adding activity. (See Activity Log Chapter 12)
- Continue your current level of Maintenance activity daily then start adding some additional daily activity you can easily achieve e.g., slow deep breathing exercises.
- Prioritize, Timetable and Reserve energy for the Micro-Rehab sessions.
- Learn the "Rest" part of the rest/activity dance. If anxiety persists, try the Defuse the Loop strategies in Chapter 15.
- Remember to pace not push.
- Tune into your body's effort levels and aim to build from a 4 to a 7 on the Rating of Perceived Exertion (RPE) scale.
- If you are bedbound start with passive movements and core work under the guidance of a physiotherapist.
- Timetable twice weekly strengthening resistance exercises and gentle stretching (well within one's energy envelope). (E.g., yellow resistance bands, light weights etc.)
- After 4 weeks of strengthening alone, introduce sub-maximal aerobic exercise (e.g., stationary foot cycling, walking, cycling, swimming) second daily.
- Have aerobic indoor options for bad weather days. E.g., foot cycle or stationary bicycle. For people with NIH or POTS consider using a reclined bicycle, rowing machine and/or Pilates Reformer.
- STOP! Begin and End all exercise sessions with mindful relaxation or meditation (the rest /activity dance) – See Appendix 5 & 6.
- Consolidate, then build your program gently every 2 to 4 weeks using the RPE and HR monitor as your guides.
- If having a bad day, consider reducing (e.g., halving) your program for that day or rescheduling it until you feel able.
- Whether or not walking is your activity of choice, by measuring your daily steps a pedometer can be a useful way to monitor overall progress and/or guide progression. Another method would be to increase your distance (includes returning to home base) by adding a distance of say, one more electric power pole or house every 2 to 4 weeks while walking outside.
- Keep a diary/journal of your program and progress. This could be combined with your Activity log.

Table Keys to Micro-Rehab

Katie's Story

Katie was an 18-year-old high school student who was referred to me by her local GP. Three years previously she had developed ME/CFS following a nasty bout of glandular fever (Epstein Barr Virus (EBV)). Prior to this she had been a sporty, bright teenager.

Her supportive family took her to numerous practitioners. Intravenous vitamin C was initially helpful but lost its effectiveness. A variety of other vitamins and supplements were tried without any benefit. Graded exercise under the guidance of an exercise physiologist gave her some minor improvement.

Katie was taking Ritalin (methylphenidate) to improve her poor concentration and she was also treated by a psychologist with Cognitive Behavioral Therapy (CBT) for an anxiety disorder, but this did little to improve her ME/CFS. It had become too difficult for her to attend school, so her mother, Trish, a secondary school teacher, home-schooled Katie, with input from the school. Katie also received permission to complete her VCE (final high school years) over three years rather than the usual two. This was her final year.

When I first met her, she was sleeping in my waiting room. I discovered this was not unusual as she was sleeping 16 hours a day and rarely leaving home. Behind her drowsiness however, Katie was a highly motivated young person and determined to get well. She wanted to do well in her VCE and go on to university studies.

Initially, I focused my treatment strategy on reducing her hours of sleep, teaching her to meditate and some cognitive techniques (we'll explore these in Chapter 15). It became clear progress was going to be slow and I felt she urgently needed as many terrain changing inputs as possible to she give her a shot at getting her life back.

CHAPTER 14 GO... GENTLY! THE REST/ACTIVITY DANCE

After discussing this with Trish and Katie, I referred her to Dr Lionel Lubitz, a pediatrician at the Austin Hospital in Melbourne, who at that time supervised a one-month inpatient rehabilitation program for teenagers suffering from ME/CFS.[4,5] This was the only intensive inpatient program for ME/CFS funded by Medicare in Australia. It could only be accessed by schoolchildren with the condition. As Katie was still at school, she was eligible and keen to grasp the opportunity.

The main focus of this program was strict bed-time routines, individually tailored rehab exercise with weekends off. Other aspects of the program included support with schoolwork, dietary advice emphasizing a low GI diet, pacing and CBT (which Katie was offered, but declined). Meals were provided, and the structured days included rest and study times.

At her first consultation after completing this month-long program the most obvious thing was that Katie was awake! Much more physically upright and alert, it was a Katie I hadn't met before. She'd found the four weeks very difficult, especially the first two weeks. Despite experiencing significant muscle pain, delated onset muscle soreness (DOMS), for the initial three weeks, with some help from doses of paracetamol, she participated fully in the individualized exercise program set out for her. The muscle pain eased in the final week.

She confided that participation in the program with other similarly challenged teenagers had helped her to stick with it. She lost an excess 2.5 kg (6 lbs.) and had renewed stamina and strength. Crucially, her sleep patterns had normalized. She was now sleeping from 10:00 p.m. to 7:00 a.m. with no daytime sleeps. Fatigue and poor concentration were much improved but still ongoing problems, along with the anxiety that went with her VCE exam study pressures, but she'd clearly turned a corner. As Tori observed, it was as if sleeping beauty had awoken and was ready to follow her dreams rather than remain in them.

Over the next six months, Katie had one significant relapse in which her fatigue levels led her to sleep during the day once again. This was related to study pressures and anxiety and an inability to focus on a textbook for more than five minutes at a time. Working on pacing strategies in relation to study, reinforcing the lessons she had learnt at the Austin, and introducing some brief mindfulness exercises helped out here.

She received special consideration and was allowed rest breaks during her exams. A high achiever, Katie performed well and gained entry into her first university preference, Forensic Science. She deferred the year, preferring to focus on continuing to improve her health and stamina before entering university.

During this year she discovered she was unable to cope with a full-time sales job but managed a half-time position. Ongoing issues of anxiety continued, and she recognized the need for structure and to address boredom. Her social life was expanding and now included a boyfriend and a driver's license. Her health now allowed her to attend a gym three times a week.

Ritalin continued to assist her ability to concentrate but she discontinued this after two years, feeling she was becoming lazy relying on the drug. In its place she trained her brain to concentrate whilst studying by setting an alarm, initially at five-minutes before taking a five-minute break. With discipline, each week she would increase the study time by one minute until she successfully achieved a 20-minute concentration span; neuroplasticity in action!

When I spoke to Katie **five years later**, I discovered that she'd remained well, was in the final year of her degree and

CHAPTER 14 GO… GENTLY! THE REST/ACTIVITY DANCE

had travelled recently overseas on her own for three months. She now attends a gym with her mother five times a week and still finds pacing important. She has recognized that if she has two or more late nights in a row, she begins to experience flulike post-exertional malaise again, so she sticks to a pretty healthy life routine. The only downside to her health has been the recent onset of Irritable Bowel Syndrome, which is responding well to a Low FODMAP (Fermentable Oligo-Di-Monosaccharides and Polyols) diet.[6]

One compelling question that arises from Katie's story, is how did she not develop severe post-exertional malaise (PEM) during such an intensive rehabilitation exercise program at the Austin? I can't be certain, but I propose two possibilities. Firstly, Katie's program was carefully structured and individualized, starting where she was able to begin and including effectively a rest/activity dance schedule with timetabled rests. Secondly, during such a supported live-in program with her peers, all her energy could be devoted to the rehabilitation process. Energy for food preparation, household chores, transport and shopping were not required, hence her energy envelope was not excessively exceeded, if at all, as it might appear at first glance. There is research evidence that concurs with this. When household activities are taken care of and there is a supportive structure for the person affected by ME/CFS, their energy levels can improve, and fatigue lessen.[6] Hence, if you are able to negotiate mini-restorative breaks as part of your work, this will increase the likelihood of maintaining a job. At the very least introducing your own regular belly breath breaks will help (See Appendix 5).

Let me emphasize again that Katie's program was skillfully designed by a multidisciplinary team, including an exercise physiologist experienced with ME/CFS. There were designated times for rest in between exercise sessions and strict bedtime routines.

[Note: The Austin hospital now offer an eight-week outpatient program for adults with ME/CFS over 18 years of age.[7] https://www.austin.org.au/Adult_CFS]

How much recovery can one expect?

Having experienced this type of rehab myself and read and witnessed my patients, like Katie, turn their ship around it is clearly possible to use this approach to assist in 'life-recovery.' What is impossible to predict is exactly how it will impact on any individual's particular situation. As I've said before we do not know why around 5% of people with ME/CFS completely recover and why 40% improve.[8-10] We do know the sooner you stop pushing and learn to pace your life the more chance you'll give your body to restore.

You do not have to be an athlete to benefit from Micro-Rehab. The gentle rebuilding of physical condition through self-awareness (guided by RPE and HR), throughout one's rehabilitation using the rest/activity dance, allows you to do this safely and provides the right conditions for the body to move towards improvement.

Other than the important effect of reversing deconditioning, Alastair Lynch, Samantha Miller, Katie, myself and others, whilst hopeful, could not have predicted the exact level of benefit to their ME/CFS we would receive when we began our rehabilitation programs.

Now that you know what it can do and that it can be safely trialed under experienced supervision, you can see why I strongly advise people to give it a shot.

CHAPTER 14 GO... GENTLY! THE REST/ACTIVITY DANCE

**Chapter 14
Key Points**

✓ Go Gently. It's OK to win your health back the slowly.
✓ See Table 1 Keys to Micro-rehab summary.
✓ Katies inspiring story.

Chapter 15
DEFUSE THE LOOP

"We can use our pain - emotional or physical - as a catalyst to begin healing not curing. To me curing means only getting back to the way we were before we became diseased. Healing is when we use our pain or illness as a catalyst to begin transforming our lives - healing our inner pain and our relationships, our hearts and our souls."

DR DEAN ORNISH, CARDIOLOGIST

Prior to developing ME/CFS, I was a medical doctor (GP) and university lecturer with a special interest in how the mind and body interact.[1] Although our understanding is still in its infancy, we are gradually discovering that many illnesses of a physical nature can be assisted by enlisting the mind as part of the treatment. I will teach you some ways to do in this chapter.

Why is this important? In any chronic illness, there tends to be an inner struggle, a struggle that if left unchecked leads to anxiety that can place added strain on an already sick body. In ME/CFS this is especially so. The illness itself is caused by a very real physical brain inflammation triggered, most commonly, by a post-viral autoimmune response *(See A Doctor's Journey back to Health Ch 5, 10-12)*. This response also leads to an overactive sympathetic nervous system that begins in the brain and among other things makes one feel anxious and hypervigilant.

The reality of Long Covid and its potential to leave a percentage of its sufferers with ME/CFS is having an impact on how society views the seriousness of ME/CFS but there is a long way to go. The combination of dealing with a serious disease in addition to a society just emerging from an outright denial of its existence, continues to be very taxing for many and we now know this stress in itself can have a negative feedback loop that aggravates the brain inflammation. The good news is, with mind-body techniques we can reverse some of this.

I am acutely aware that in relation to ME/CFS recommending any psychological/mind-body treatment is a touchy subject. You'll recall that in *A Doctor's Journey Back to Health Chapters 2 and 13,* I presented the history of the illness and the bizarre circumstances in which it came to be falsely attributed to being all in a person's 'head.' Attempts to psychologize treatment based upon this false premise have been extremely damaging. As a counterpunch this has led some people with ME/CFS to avoid psychological strategies altogether, preferring to stick with biomedical treatments, none of whom at this time make much difference. This is unfortunate; yet given the history of this cursed disease, understandable. I ask you to put all that aside for now and utilize whatever help you can.

Let me teach you simple techniques that can help you not only cope better and enjoy your life more, but also may improve the condition itself as it would any neurological disorder.

Neurons that Fire Together Wire Together

The techniques I'll share in this chapter have the potential to both reduce anxiety and to rewire destructive patterns. What do I mean by rewire? It is possible, as we now know from functional Magnetic Resonance Imaging (fMRI) research that brain structures, if subject to repeated positive inputs, can physically alter. Inputs such as problem solving, meditation and psychotherapy have been demonstrated to change/build new pathways within days or weeks.[2-7]

This may explain my observation as to why some people with ME/

CFS who commit to these strategies every day can see improvements within weeks. More research is needed, but it seems possible that this rewiring process may also reduce the brain inflammation initiated by the triggering viral illness. For instance, we know that inflammation of the prefrontal cortex (a part of the brain) along with the loss of brain cells (grey matter) reverses after the successful treatment of chronic pain.[8]

Before we delve into specific strategies a proviso; some people will need more psychological support than the approaches outlined here. As I myself needed years ago, some of you may need ongoing psychotherapy. Even so, these strategies are safe and can assist any formal counselling process.

Defusing the Hypervigilance Loop

Until pacing is mastered, the unpredictability of post-exertional malaise (PEM) means you can no longer trust your body. This can play havoc with one's sanity. In addition, it has been postulated (the Kindling hypothesis) that at least in a subset of people affected by ME/CFS, an immune system response (e.g., triggered by an infection and/or the constant feeling of being under threat of crashing), **sensitizes** the brain's limbic (emotional) system which communicates with the hypothalamic-pituitary-adrenal (HPA) axis, so **that even a slight worry can trigger an energy sapping, disproportionate, physiological stress response**.[9-11]

Under the influence of this Central Nervous System (CNS) malfunction you lose trust in your body, without necessarily being aware of it, and you can find yourself worrying about symptoms and whether you will overdo it with activities. This hypervigilance can magnify problems many times over. Repetitive worrying can occur in the form of *conscious or unconscious* thoughts, such as: 'Oh no, I've over done it again!'

'I might crash!'

'How will I cope?' These may be valid concerns worthy of problem-solving, but not useful things to dwell on over and over again. When this repetitive-thinking does happen, it can push the 'fight or flight' sympathetic nervous system and HPA axis into overdrive, constantly triggering the release of chemicals such as adrenaline, noradrenaline and cortisol. The chronic ongoing release of these chemicals can weaken the immune system and further aggravate symptoms such as fatigue, sleep problems and muscle pain.[12]

This consequent worsening of symptoms can then trigger further worrying thoughts, stimulating the fight or flight response again, keeping the negative feedback loop spiraling on and on to the point of exhaustion. In my clinical experience, if this is recognized and dealt with it can speed improvement. Whereas if it goes unrecognized it can become a significant illness perpetuating factor which can lead some people to avoiding most activities altogether. This inevitably leads to further physical deconditioning and frailty.

Fortunately, this CNS sensitization, where even a harmless noise can trigger a stress/threat response, can be dampened, and the hypervigilance loop disrupted using mind-body therapies.

Defuse the Loop: Problem Solving

With ME/CFS there can be a lot of annoying problems that can be easily solved once identified. These can range from needing a straw to help you to drink, to getting other household members to quieten down, to having a meal sorted.

The first step is admitting this to yourself and then involving others in nutting out solution(s). Making a 'What Cheeses me off' list can help clarify things for all. You might consider occasionally placing it next to your daily 0-10 rating score (see Ch 5). Making this list can be therapeutic and alert others to your needs. Just don't expect them all to be solved at once.

The Drummer

I remember a neighbor who would start practicing on his drums any time of day and sometimes night. It really used to upset me, especially as I found myself worrying he might start at any time, even when he wasn't playing. Just anticipating when he would break my quiet time was getting to me as inevitably it seemed to happen when I was trying to meditate or rest. So, I asked a friend to knock on his door, explain my situation and get his phone number for me. We spoke on the phone and I explained my story further. He agreed to practice only between certain hours.

He broke the time 'rules' a few times and it took a few more calls before he got the routine, but because we'd made a connection and I had his number to call if needed I wasn't as stressed. I had some boundaries around my space. This example highlights one of the keys to managing stress - having or creating a sense of control over your immediate environment; be it sounds, smells, access to food and water etc.

Pacing also helps to regulate your energy levels and gives you a greater sense of control over your symptoms. These safer conditions then allow you to work on your inner sense of equilibrium.

I emphasize again that you may need help from a counsellor to develop your inner self-worth and/or communication skills in order to establish healthy boundaries. Sometimes the hardest boundaries to make are with our nearest and dearest.

Mindfulness

Calming the mind and body with conscious slow deep breaths along with mindfulness meditation or relaxation (see Appendix 5 and 6) is a good place to start defusing the inner stress pattern. If you have not done so yet, go to Appendix 5 and try it. Then pick one of the three exercises in Appendix 6 and have a go. Once you find an exercise that suits you then make it a daily practice.

The mindfulness process will also help you to become more aware of unhelpful circulating thoughts so that you can identify and resolve them. This may also require assistance from a counsellor or psychologist, ideally experienced with ME/CFS. Some of these services are available online. There are other approaches you can try on your own and we will expand on these in a moment.

Cognitive Behavioral Therapy (CBT)

Based upon a false belief that ME/CFS was a psychiatric not biomedical disease, CBT was for decades a recommended treatment for ME/CFS. The National Institute for Health and Care Excellence (NICE) in the UK recently reframed CBT in the context of a "supportive psychological therapy which aims to improve wellbeing and quality of life"[13] and **not** as a cure. Hence NICE also does not recommend psychological programs like the Lightening Process or other psychological based cure-alls. Rather they suggest these psychological offerings should be seen in the same light as CBT, potentially supportive therapies.

My experience and approach is a little more nuanced than this as anything that can defuse the loop of anxiety and thus clarify one's true perception can improve one's effectiveness at Micro-Rehab.

Some people who'd sought my help had not benefited from CBT but did benefit from other mind-body approaches. But mind your wallet as they can be pricey!

CHAPTER 15 DEFUSE THE LOOP

What's Involved?

Psychologists trained in Cognitive Behavioral Therapy (CBT) emphasize the role of thinking and its impact on how a person feels and acts. Classic CBT involves identifying unhelpful ruminating thoughts like 'I'll never get well' and disputing their validity by asking yourself "what evidence do I have that this thought is true?"

My experience is that CBT in the hands of a psychologist familiar with ME/CFS thought patterns can be brilliant. But if unfamiliar with the specific challenges a person with ME/CFS faces, is as useful a tool as a butter knife is in attempting to slice a loaf of crusty bread. Not completely useless, but not great!

By contrast when one becomes aware of the specific symptom thoughts that can predominate in the thinking of someone with ME/CFS, the butter knife grows some teeth. For example, thoughts such as 'what if I never get better?' And 'nothing I do makes any difference.' If you are familiar with the patterns of thinking like this that occur with ME/CFS (See Appendix 7 for further examples) CBT can help you to recognize what's real fear and what's overblown fear.

Ultimately mindfulness with CBT brings an awareness of one's unhelpful thinking so that it can be challenged, and the hypervigilance loop defused, reducing the intensity of the thoughts which can help reduce symptoms by calming the brain's alarm system (in the HPA axis in the brainstem).

CBT is the most well-researched method of treatment for ME/CFS. Cochrane reviews, considered the gold standard in clinical research circles, have demonstrated it is helpful,[14,15] but as I've alluded to, there is controversy. Rather than spending too much time on the origin of this controversy here, I've devoted a chapter to it in my previous book, *A Doctor's Journey Back to Health Ch 13*.

My clinical experience with this, is that whilst CBT can be helpful, specific psychological therapies designed for ME/CFS can be even more effective. Don't get me wrong, CBT can be invaluable but its approach tends to be generic, applicable to a wide range of illnesses. Not that this is a problem, but sometimes you need to add even more ME/CFS-specific teeth to that butter knife.

Other mind-body therapies

Fortunately, there are other mind-body therapies inspired and developed with ME/CFS in mind to help to defuse the hypervigilance loop. Three that I am familiar with are: Gupta Amygdala Retraining,[16,17] which incorporates a particular thought stopping technique, visualization and meditation; Mickel therapy,[18] which focuses more on being aware of one's feelings, learning to identify the need for boundaries and how to create them, acting positively and proactively to restore one's feeling of safety and well-being; and the Lightening Process which has intensive three-day workshops (beyond the energy capacity and wallet-size of many people with ME/CFS) that help people to recognize self-defeating patterns of thinking and replace them with empowering ones. As I've said, if you choose to go with one of these, check your budget.

While unlike CBT, which has solid research to back its usefulness in ME/CFS, these three techniques lack adequate scientific research to back the claims they make. However, their principle components are sound and some of my patients have benefited greatly from them. However, just as not everyone will respond to CBT, not everyone will be suited to Gupta, Mickel or the Lightening Process either. Another useful website that focuses on these and similar techniques is https://ansrewire.com/

Like CBT, all of these techniques are potentially beneficial if committed to and practiced. Recall that positive neuroplasticity demands repetition with frequent, persistent practice to achieve long term results.

Let me share one final approach that integrates many of these ideas. It is one I've created myself and many people who consulted me with ME/CFS found helpful.

Replace your Automatic Negative Thoughts (ANTS) with Positive Emotional Thoughts (PETS)

Apart from **disputing** unhelpful ruminating thoughts via CBT (e.g., by asking yourself "what evidence do I have that this thought is true?") or **disrupting** them by thought stopping (e.g., flicking a rubber band around one's wrist every time unhelpful thinking is noticed), one can also try **replacing** thoughts. Let me explain.

An approach that I developed with my patients and which you could use right now, is to replace your ANTS with PETS. If you look at Appendix 7, you'll see there is a list of automatic negative thoughts (ANTS) which I have modified from Gupta's work. Without exception, every person affected by ME/CFS that I saw could relate to at least one category of these ANTS. Some of these thoughts need to be acknowledged, addressed and acted upon, but as I've explained, ruminating over these and creating the problems of the hypervigilance loop is unnecessary and harmful.

One way of challenging these automatic negative thoughts (ANTS) is with PETS. I'm not talking about cats or dogs here, although they could help too! Here a PET is a Positive Emotional Thought, that is, any thought that you say to yourself that leaves you **feeling** better. The emphasis here is on feeling; whether that be upliftment or just relief. This usually differs from affirmations, positive things that you tell yourself, in that it is only a PET if it makes you feel better. If it feels forced, you're on the wrong track. Note that a PET is a very personal thing and what works for you may not work for someone else. Here are a few examples from people with ME/CFS who tried this:

'It's okay. It's not an emergency.'

'I don't have to solve it all today.'

'This too will pass.'

'Even though I am unable to work, I love and accept myself.' I've listed further examples my patients have come up with in Appendix 7 to give you the idea. Remember though, one person's PET may be another person's ANT. So, don't be surprised if you find some of these examples annoying. Generally, the best PET is one you come up with intuitively or read, that causes an inner comforting sigh.

A Defusing Plan

Week 1

- For one week, start each day with some slow deep breathing then a 5 minute mindfulness meditation before breakfast.
- See if you can identify your most common ANTS. Jot these down. If any PETS come to you in this time jot these down also. You may find some of these PETS arise in direct response to and act as an antidote for the ANTS.
- If you are struggling to identify your ANTS you could try the 'morning pages' exercise (see further on in this chapter) and see if any examples arise.
- If you are still unable to come up with any check out Appendix 7 and see if any ring true.

Week 2

- Continue with your daily deep breathing and morning mindfulness meditation. Add an evening 5 minute meditation to this regime before dinner.
- Look out for ANTS and record these.
- Try coming up with some PETS and record these.

CHAPTER 15 DEFUSE THE LOOP

> **Week 3**
> - Continue your week 2 program.
> - When you notice ANTS arising - dispute, disrupt or replace these ANTS with PETS. Repeat this regularly throughout the day especially whenever you notice yourself ruminating on ANTS.
> - Combine your 'PET talk' with slow deep belly breath pauses. Then meditate again in the evening.
> - Towards the end of the evening meditation time bring into your mind an image of a healthier, happier you. Do this in as much detail as you are able (a past memory of a healthier time may help). For example, you might like to visualize yourself standing strong on a beautiful beach. Feel the warmth of the sun on your back, hear the sounds of the waves rolling into shore, smell the salty air, feel strong in your body. Like a PET, the aim of this mind-body exercise is to feel good. Once you achieve this, anchor this feeling by pressing together your right thumb and forefinger (in an okay symbol). You can now use this reassuring symbol any time of day, for example, every time you stop and belly breath and/or use a PET. You may even find it counteracts an ANT on its own.
>
> Be determined and persistent and you will succeed. However, if your ANTS prove recalcitrant, you may need some guidance with this or to take a different approach. Do not be disheartened, its often just a matter of finding what works best for you.

PETS Used By Date

You may find that some PETS lose their effectiveness over time, so you may need to keep coming up with new ones. Sometimes you strike gold and a PET maintains its benefits for months. Be creative, anything goes and once you come up with some effective ones, jot them down and use them whenever it feels natural to you to break the unhelpful hypervigilance pattern and defuse the loop.

Julie's Story

I first consulted with 21-year-old Julie eight months after she was diagnosed with glandular fever. Prior to falling ill, she was studying Interior Design at University four-days a week and working in a retail store twice a week. Getting to University or to work would involve at least two hours of driving each day. She also attended a gym two to three times per week.

As the year progressed, she had increasing episodes of pharyngitis (inflamed sore throat) but tests did not reveal that the glandular fever had returned. By the time she consulted with me she was too unwell to attend either university or work and could barely cope with a 5-minute walk, let alone attend the gym. Her symptoms included profound fatigue, post-exertional malaise, unrefreshing altered sleep (14 hours in bed/day), muscle pain (predominantly in her legs), diminished concentration abilities and autonomic dysfunction with dizziness and difficulty with prolonged standing. She had to move from her shared rental apartment back into her family home so that her mother could care for her basic needs.

After introducing the concept and importance of pacing to Julie, her management turned to optimizing her sleep patterns. She was going to bed at 9.00 pm, but it would take three hours for her to fall asleep and if she awoke during the night it would take her hours to get back to sleep again. It would be midday or later before she arose. A relaxation audio and a small dose of the medication amitriptyline markedly improved her sleep patterns (falling to sleep within 15 minutes and sleeping 10 or 11 hours).

I also referred Julie to an exercise physiologist to obtain an appropriate individualized Micro-Rehab home-based exercise program. This was complemented by a low GI diet which included frequent two hourly snacks. She knew a nutritionist she was happy to consult with who

CHAPTER 15 DEFUSE THE LOOP

helped her with this. Julie was also someone who enjoyed a drink, having six alcoholic drinks a night if she was out at a social event. I explained this was not a helpful or healthy habit and when she was well enough again to even contemplate socializing and drinking alcohol, to limit it to a maximum of one drink in any 24-hr period.

Julie was diligent and determined to do whatever she could to overcome her health problems. It became clear that she was trapped in the hypervigilance loop and that anxiety was a significant barrier. I introduced her to slow belly breathing, mindfulness meditation and got her to identify her automatic negative thoughts (ANTS). She dealt with these using thought stopping (disrupting) and counteracting them with positive emotional thoughts (PETS), like, 'my body is resilient,' regularly many times each day. Her anxiety abated, and she felt more energetic. Note: Nowadays I would also have prescribed CBD oil (see Chapter 4) for Julie to assist her with anxiety.

Following this program Julie's strength and stamina gradually and steadily improved. She had several setbacks along the way with worsening symptoms all associated with pharyngitis (sore throat) and enlarged lymph glands in her neck. Nonetheless, after six months she considered herself to be 90% recovered. She was now getting a good night's sleep without the need for amitriptyline, was continuing a home-based exercise program as well as attending a Pilates class twice a week. In addition to this, she was now swimming gentle laps at the local pool and was able to stand for hours at a time without the need to sit down. She felt confident she would be able to return to her studies the following year and in the meantime, was planning a trip to London to visit her sister.

I asked Julie to share what she felt were the keys to her restoration. I'll list these for you in her words:

- The need to be organized and establish a healthy routine.

- Prioritizing what's most important. In making life decisions think about how this will affect me and ask myself 'does this feel right?'
- Don't push. Pace and stop when tired.
- A balanced lifestyle: sleeping well, eating healthily and regularly, exercising, meditation and deep breathing and drinking more water.
- Aim to go to bed early and wake up earlier, doing my best to stick to the routine.
- Keeping my exercise levels sub-maximal, monitoring my RPE and heart rate.
- Recognize that there are more things to enjoy than just going out on weekends and drinking alcohol. Hanging out with friends, cooking and reading for instance.
- Identifying my previous life was out of balance with too much work and travel time.
- Using Positive Emotional Thoughts (PETS), like telling myself, 'Every day I am closer to recovering from CFS.'
- Respect the fact that when I fall sick, I need adequate time to recover.
- Don't take University or work etc. so seriously (don't sweat the small stuff).
- Choose my friends carefully.

Defuse the Loop: Problem Solving

If you can relate to some of the things in Julie's list that are of concern to you it can be very useful to apply a problem-solving approach to them. You could start by writing them down or saying them out loud, even if only to yourself. Just being honest enough to name stuff can help. List them and have a go at addressing them one by one either on your own or with a friend or counsellor.

CHAPTER 15 DEFUSE THE LOOP

In tougher times, Tori and I found social workers and financial counsellors were particularly helpful for problem solving issues in the management of our day to day life. A good way to start is to list the pros and cons of different solutions and identify the specifics of your problem/s at hand. It can be surprising how much identifying and addressing the problems in your life can defuse anxiety.

A Caution

I have had several patients whom I taught to defuse their hypervigilance loop who very quickly noticed an increase in their energy levels (some immediately), like Caitlin (see Ch 10). So excited were they, that they stopped pacing. After several days like this they crashed and were in a worse state for weeks. The message here is that energy liberation is possible but has to be handled in a carefully paced way. My advice is to continue pacing, put any extras in the reserve bank, gradually building activity levels and restoring enough physical conditioning so that any new-found energy can be contained and sustained.

Feeling Trapped

Deeper psychological and/or interpersonal issues can be a contributing trigger and an ongoing issue for some people with any chronic illness including ME/CFS. For example, some patients reported to me that they initially contracted the illness when they had excessive responsibilities, or when they had multiple work and personal stressors from which there appeared to be no way out. Feeling trapped in a job you don't want to do is another example of this.

This is a recipe for a breakdown (some call it adrenal burnout), for susceptibility to ME/CFS, autoimmune disease or a mental health issue. Finding a way through this in a way that breaks the pattern that allowed it to occur in the first place, may require considerable support and psychotherapy. This psychological pattern is often linked with feeling driven.

Interpersonal Challenges

As difficult as this topic is to address, people with ME/CFS can find that one of their major challenges is dealing with the people in their lives. Sometimes it may even be challenging to relate to the people or person who is caring for you. Some of the issues that may arise can be due to the levels of understanding and believability of the illness. It is hoped that this book may be one possible avenue for educating yourself and those around you. Other sources of educational material are ME/CFS support groups and the ME/CFS society in your state.

Other common issues are related to the effects of the illness itself. As I've mentioned earlier, people with the condition can be highly sensitized to noise, smells, light and activity in their environment. They can also be travelling at a very slow rhythm compared with the rest of society and find that others in their circle or their household are travelling at a much faster rate. This may cause the person with the illness to feel stressed and unable to cope. This is no one's fault but it can be valuable to identify and to problem solve any issues arising out of a difference in pace and needs. Again, social workers can be very valuable people to consult in relation to these lifestyle matters. One technique that I've already shared at the end of Chapter 5 is the daily scorecard/emoji to let people know how you are feeling from 1 to 10 without the need for further explanation. And if you are not comfortable sharing this information then consider it for own self-awareness.

Sometimes interpersonal problems run very deep and further psychotherapy is required to address this.

CHAPTER 15 DEFUSE THE LOOP

Feeling Driven

Not everyone with a driven personality will end up with ME/CFS, but if it is part of what leads to the problem then it may need extra attention as it can fuel the loop and drain vital energy. People I recognized were driven characters, like myself, whom I consulted with and who had ME/CFS, benefitted from more intensive psychotherapy to address childhood patterns of behavior and thinking as part of their restoration. This drive to succeed and prove oneself can be insatiable and can lead to a disconnection between the signals one's body is giving to stop and rest and the mind's desire to continue pushing. The challenge for these people, ultimately, is to learn to self-soothe, parent and love oneself, regardless of other's opinions. Only then can the art of pacing be fully integrated.

This can require considerable reflection and counselling as the origin of this driven feeling often lies in family dynamics and patterns developed in childhood. Understanding these origins and becoming aware of this unhealthy, pushy pattern can allow one to choose not to follow it anymore, establishing a more self-aware, self-accepting, balanced approach to life in its place.

Childhood Trauma – Complex PTSD (Post traumatic stress disorder)

There is a subset of people with ME/CFS who have experienced significant trauma and a lack of love and/or safety in their childhoods. While the strategies presented in this chapter for defusing the loop may still be useful for these people, additional supportive and possibly in-depth therapy may be needed to assist the restoration process as the hypervigilance of the fight-flight system has been set on an extremely high level, making clarity in paced rehab very difficult until this deep trauma is acknowledged and worked with.

Morning Pages

One way I found useful for myself and my patients in helping them to safely vent anger and other built up emotions was morning pages. I learnt this technique from Julia Cameron's book *The Artist's Way*.[19] It involves stream of consciousness writing. Essentially, soon after waking, you write whatever comes into your head onto a pad. Anything goes for a few minutes, swear words, telling people off, railing at society, whatever; all is encouraged ('blurts' Julia refers to them as.)

After a few minutes of connecting to your feelings and letting them rip, you stop. Tear out the sheets of paper you've just written on and tear them to shreds or burn them i.e., make them indecipherable. This exercise is not for show and tell, it is just to help you get stuff off your chest. That's it.

Like micro-rehab, take it gently as while cathartic it can be taxing. So I recommend timeouts to integrate new levels of understanding and to recoup in the form of days off delving. I suggest do it every second morning for 10 days, then decide if you wish to continue it, and if so, how often.

See https://juliacameronlive.com/basic-tools/morning-pages/

Self Compassion

When things get really tough there is one strategy that seems too gentle to make a difference, yet does. In my own situation I'd be come a bit of a grump and not very pleasant to be around. So obsessed with finding answers to my situation was I, that I'd forgotten to live in the now. To change this pattern, I had to actively reclaim my kinder self and my sense of humor by looking on the funny side of everyday life. I soon realized my nearest and dearest were better off and so was I!

Later I would discover the work of Christopher Germer and Kristin

CHAPTER 15 DEFUSE THE LOOP

Neff. Kristin's book, *Self Compassion*,[20,21] helped me to anchor the conscious efforts I'd developed myself. The four steps that she suggests you use when facing any struggle are:

1. Acknowledge to yourself that this is a moment of suffering.
2. Know that other people in the world are experiencing similar suffering (you are not alone).
3. Place your hands gently on your chest and say to yourself, "may I hold my suffering with tenderness and kindness."
4. Say to yourself, "may I give myself the compassion that I need."

I find this approach helps me in tough moments to nurture myself and paradoxically stay open to others. Kristin's research has shown that people who practice self-compassion can more sustainably be compassionate towards others, that is, they are less likely to experience compassion fatigue. If you are struggling with this, then you might like to try it. It combines beautifully with the *Soften and Flow* meditation (see Appendix 6).

A Physical Illness

The effect of the mind on health and disease can be huge. Our health education systems like to separate physical and mental health, in doing so this can limit possible benefits of a more holistic treatment approach.

Nonetheless it is important to remember research confirms that ME/CFS is a physical neurological disorder. As Tori and I revealed in *A Doctor's Journey Back to Health*, IT IS REAL! I felt at times during my illness that if I could only get to the bottom of my emotional problems that my illness would be cured. In fact, in time I did get to the bottom of most of my major emotional and interpersonal issues but lo and behold the illness was still there! I believed the false publicity that ME/

CFS was a psychological disease as this is what I had been taught. I was wrong.

However, until we have more specific treatments, all aspects of the terrain, be they more inner psychological as this chapter has addressed, or more obvious physical, like social support, pacing, Micro-Rehab, diet, sleep etc, need to be attended to if you are to have the best shot at significant improvement.

Chapter 15
Key Points

✓ The hypervigilance loop refers to the inappropriate activation of the HPA axis.
✓ In ME/CFS this pathway is most commonly activated by a viral infection triggering an autoimmune response that leads to brains inflammation. Apart from all of the other symptoms of ME/CFS (see Appendix 1), this commonly presents itself as ruminating automatic negative thoughts (ANTS).
✓ After settling the sympathetic nervous system (e.g., with relaxation/meditation) one can become aware of this pattern of rumination.
✓ Once this is clearly identified it can be dealt with by specific mind-body techniques that either: settle, dispute, thought stop/disrupt; or replace ANTS with PETS.
This has the potential to rewire the destructive thinking patterns with healthier ones and reduce anxiety.
✓ We know from fMRI research, that brain structures can be physically changed by psychological techniques like: problem solving, mindfulness, meditation, CBT and psychotherapy. This process may also reduce the brain inflammation found in ME/CFS, thus not only helping one's psyche but also physical symptoms as well.

Chapter 16
RUTH CIRCA 2022

Forteen years on since we met her in 2008, housebound with her dog Jaco (see Chapter 1), I asked Ruth to write another essay to counterpoint, Unexpected Friendship, the essay she wrote back then. So, in Ruth's words...

Healing Notes

"I breathed in sweet relief as the sound of the bow on the strings filled my ears. I felt my heart expanding with gratitude that I could play again after an eight-year sabbatical. The music flowed through my body, like water coursing through the ocean. It filled my whole being with beautiful vibrant energy until I felt an epitome of joy, like that of the sun breaking out of the clouds on a grey day.

I turned around delighted as the surprise greeted me. My dad Rob came into the room with his newly-acquired tenor guitar, joining me with my choice of jazz tunes. As the duo of strings blended together, this was a language that I could understand, that I could express and communicate without a need for words. A language that my mind, body and spirit understood so well. My arms felt lighter than air now rather than a heavy burdened weight. I felt myself soaring; the sound reverberated throughout the kitchen and rose up to meet the high ceiling dome of the room. There is nothing quite like it in the world, the dialogue between two instruments. We both knew what a blessing it was to be able to play together once more.

I'd been clasped by the black clutches of illness for many years forcing me into a paralysis. I'd yearned to pick up my beautiful violin from my great grandmother, to hear myself play the resonant sounds.

There's nothing quite like having strings under my fingers and feeling the vibrations of the strings throughout my body. Surprisingly my dormant period had not made me too much the worse for wear. I'd always considered this period of dormancy a prison but perhaps it was what I'd needed, what my body had needed; to rest so that I could fully appreciate the gift that music could bring.

This luxury of playing, a sandstone of my identity had been brutally stripped from me, in the cruellest fashion. The grief had been unbearable; playing music had always been part of my life. I had learnt to sing before I had learnt to speak at nine months of age; my first song had been a Jewish hymn Dai Dai Anu. Ever since I could remember I always had an instrument under my fingers. From age 6, I played piano and then took up violin at the age of 10.

After I was struck down by ME/CFS the ease and accessibility of music suddenly became a foreign concept for I had no more energy to put into these pleasures. What had been a joy, effortless, had become a strain, draining me of the precious life force energy that I needed for survival.

I'll never forget the feeling of the onset, as if a ton of bricks had been laid upon my body. Every movement had felt like an enormous effort. Lifting up my arms for any length of time to hold my violin had been impossible. How blissfully different life was now. The ease of movement, the lightness in my limbs was heaven compared with the impossibly oppressed, heavy, restricted and sluggish body I had experienced. I reflected on the years of rehab I had done, and am still doing, diligently going to the pilates gym, to rebuild the muscle strength I had lost. I need to point out how crucial this upper body training has been to enable me to use my arms once again to sustain a violin hold. The endurance of playing had been too difficult initially and so I took up teaching myself guitar, as it was easier posture-wise. I now enjoy the variety of playing two stringed instruments.

CHAPTER 16 RUTH CIRCA 2022

When the wings of fatigue had settled around me, enclosing me in their strong grasp, this fundamental aspect of my being had been stolen from me. Being once more able to play has given me a new lease of life. Like reviving a flame from a withered ember.

I guess it was a natural progression, seeing as music is so innate to me, having come from a family of musicians, that I should go on to teach violin. As I reflect on the journey of the last twelve years, from being bed-bound to now teaching violin students for a few hours on a weekly basis, I am filled with awe and wonder at the body's capacity to heal.

I would never have thought this progress possible, and teaching violin has been a sustainable effort through careful pacing, monitoring and balance. It has been a wonderful way to regain a sense of independence and confidence, and to contribute to others' musical journeys. I love sharing my knowledge and have a lot of fun watching my students' progress and I enjoy being involved in the learning process. It's a special bond that is created between music teacher and student and I feel blessed to have this unique connection with each person. ME/CFS is an isolating and lonely journey and it is indeed a beautiful gift to be able to share and give to others a safe space in which to explore sound and have my own sense of self value restored.

It's extremely fulfilling to rediscover and pass on the tricks and tools I have been taught. My long-term memory allows me to draw on my past experiences and equips me with an energy requiring less effort than drawing on short-term memory.

Recalling tips from 15 years ago is very automatic because they have been etched into my subconscious mind. The hundreds of hours I had spent in my teens practising, honing my craft has paid off. I can now play easily, my mind relaxes, the playing is engrained in the cells of my body. It is a skill I will have for life. People experiencing ME/CFS are always looking for any short cuts that make life easier by using less energy.

Teaching helps me to be kinder and more compassionate to myself; I find that the gentle coaching that I offer to my students infiltrates into my own life and I am more generous with my own thoughts and feelings. I am also less judgemental of my limitations and have learnt to trust my intuition.

I've also found that the beauty of playing music and teaching is that it keeps me rooted firmly in the present moment. Any troubles I am carrying melt away as I focus clearly on the notes and how best to express these. If the mind wanders when one is playing, one cannot deliver the music in its entirety as it deserves to be heard. In this respect playing music is like an act of meditation for me. This reinforces the meditation practice I have adopted since the beginning of my ME/CFS. Meditation has been a crucial part of my daily routine and integrating my music work with this is part of also restoring my mental health

In the early years of my ME/CFS illness I felt caged; claustrophobic behind iron

bars. It was firstly through community singing that the compressed walls of my cell had widened, the lock on the door had started to loosen until gradually coming undone, and the constricted prison had slowly dissipated, finally vanishing completely. These weekly choir rehearsals have been an integral part of my life-restoration. I've made many friends through this avenue and hearing the sound of our unified voices is truly a very healing experience.

When I was too unwell to hold an instrument, being part of something bigger than myself, and feeling supported in this experience, brought me much comfort and joy. I was able to contribute to my community without being burdened by responsibility. When my voice was too weak to sing, I could enjoy being present with others in the room, the breathing component of singing was a healthy technique to adopt, and the sound of the combined voices in the room was a purely magical

CHAPTER 16 RUTH CIRCA 2022

energy pill for my ears and a soothing sensation for my cells to soak up.

Now 14 years after my diagnosis, this much-anticipated social outing and highlight of my week continues to be an incredibly powerful musical aspect of my life. It is my soul medicine. I also accompany the choir in a string trio which has been a beautiful addition to our group.

Studies have shown that our brain neurology and chemistry changes when we sing in a choir, as the neurotransmitter oxytocin is produced. This facilitates trust in others and in the world. I have also found it has instilled a greater trust in myself and a boost of my self-esteem. It reduces the feelings of isolation, anxiety and loneliness that ME/CFS can bring and replaces these with a natural, healthy choral high! My mind feels clear and more open after choir as the two hemispheres of the brain are utilized; it calms the left-brain thinking mind which is often over-working and helps integrate the right-brain feeling centre of the mind without creating feelings of overwhelm.

When Steven asked me to contribute to his second book on ME/CFS, I thought it was an ideal opportunity to illustrate the contrast between my early days of ME/CFS and the abundant life I now experience. I have tried to show this through my ability to play and experience music. While I still face challenges on a day to day basis and life is far from smooth sailing, I have become better at accepting and celebrating my achievements and my limitations with grace and focusing my energy and attention on what I can positively influence. As a result, I feel very blessed with my quality of life.

I hope that this reflection gives readers a sense of the vast improvement which is entirely possible after being incredibly unwell. May it bring hope that it is possible to regain parts of your life that you have lost."

SUMMING UP

"Failure does not tolerate persistence."
ALLAN JEANS - AUSTRALIAN RULES FOOTBALL COACH

In a society that lauds people for pushing through their limitations to succeed, having ME/CFS can be torturous. The more we push to keep up the worse it gets and the more scars it leaves. While effective specific treatments remain elusive, navigating the reality of this disease and finding a way forward requires a different approach, an approach that improves the 'terrain,' the body's self-healing systems. Let me summarize the eight keys I have suggested with these two Tables I presented in Chapter 3:

Social Support	Pacing
Restorative Sleep	Micro-Rehab - Rest/Activity Dance
Nourishing Diet	Mind-body therapies – Defuse the Loop
Appropriate Movement	Restoring body-mind trust - instinct
Table 1. FUNDAMENTAL 4 (ME/CFS plus all Chronic Illnesses)	**Table 2. SPECIFIC 4 (ME/CFS-Specific Strategies)**

More specific treatments will no doubt come to light with further research. There is however, no reason to avoid these general 'terrain-improving' measures that are already utilized successfully in the management of other neurological disorders, like Parkinson's and MS, with the proviso that they are informed and supervised in an ME/CFS-specific way. This is what I've presented in this book.

Progress

I know we covered this somewhat in Chapter 5, but it is so important that I'd like to reiterate some key points. My experience and the experience of others affected by ME/CFS is that the road to recovering a life, whether that be partial or complete, often features setbacks. It is important at these times, which can sometimes feel like you're back at square one, to remember that most people will take two steps forward and then one or even three steps backwards from time to time, and to be gentle on yourself. Using the skills shared in earlier chapters, you know now how to restore your balance and move forwards once again.

At times it can be beneficial to look back and see how far you've come, the strategies you've acquired, the things you have learned, rather than how much more you've got to go, this is where having a journal/diary can help (see Chapter 5).

In contrast to setbacks, 'set-forwards' can pose their own problems too. I have witnessed people affected by ME/CFS, like Caitlin (Chapter 10), suddenly gain in energy when they break the hypervigilance loop, for instance, or start to benefit from their Micro-Rehab. Buoyed by the feeling, they then forget about pacing, overstep their body's capacity and use all their energy up in a rush, only to crash back down again for days or weeks. Caitlin's story was a cautionary tale in this regard. The key message here is that ***pacing is just as important when you're feeling better as when you're feeling worse.*** Your body has lost muscle due to months or years of inactivity, so it needs time to catch up. The ideal is to keep pacing and gradually expand your life. Increase activity in manageable steps so that you can begin to strengthen your deconditioned body and start to build some reserves. This may be more easily said than done when you are experiencing the best energy you've felt in years. Still, this is the challenge to be confronted.

Good News

The good news is this, you will **not have to be so strict forever**. As you do gain physical condition and mental ease, your confidence and self-awareness will grow. You'll then find you respond to your body's messages on an as needs basis more and more naturally. Your energy envelope in this circumstance will continue to expand or stabilize and be less reliant on 'military precision.' and more naturally on instinct/intuition and self-mastery.

The Importance of Stories

While we need more research into the management of ME/CFS to pin down the best terrain enhancing approaches, we can read between the lines of people's stories and discover common principles. In *A Doctor's Journey Back to Health*, Tori and I shared our story, whilst here we've included other hopeful stories from our patients and from elsewhere to illustrate common threads between them all.

So, let's revisit the stories we've shared in this book and how long each person took to achieve a level of life-restoration they felt was significant following the initiation of the sort of terrain-treatment approach I've presented here:

- **Ruth Gador** took five years from being housebound to obtaining her driver's license and participating in study and part-time work teaching violin. (see Chapters 1 and 16)
- **Samantha Miller** took five years from bedbound to part-time work. (see Ch 11)

- **Steven Sommer** (myself) close to housebound when Dr Daniel Lewis knocked on my door. Three years later after 11 years of not practicing medicine, I returned to part-time medical practice and undergraduate and postgraduate teaching (see *A Doctor's Journey Back to Health*).
- **Alastair Lynch** 12 months to return to playing AFL football at the top level, albeit on a gentler training and travel regime than his teammates (see Ch 12).
- **Katie** from three years of being housebound and homeschooled to full time University study after two and a half years of paced rehab. Five years later able to tour Europe alone and complete her University degree (see Ch 14).
- **Julie**, recently diagnosed, took 10 months after dropping out of Uni and work, to return to part-time work and being able to fly to London to visit her sister. (see Ch15).

It is impossible to say how long you will need to carefully apply this terrain enhancing approach in order to achieve what you would call a significant level of life-restoration until more quality outcome-based research into programs like this one are done. But the critical thing is that others have gone before you; it is possible!

The Six Months Test

If you apply yourself to the program I've presented here with diligence, most of you will be noticing improvements within six months. If despite tweaking the program with your health practitioner, you are not improving, are worsening or are developing new symptoms then see your GP for a checkup. It is always beneficial for your GP to reassess where you're at from time to time, and to ensure nothing is being overlooked. She/he may need to revisit the diagnosis and make sure it is correct (See Appendix 1, 2 and 3). If she/he confirms a diagnosis of ME/CFS then consider these perpetuating factors as possibilities.

Potential perpetuating factors (modified from McIntyre and Valling) [1,2]

- Unable to accept the illness and allow adequate life-pacing for healing.
- Repeated overactivity, inappropriate lifestyle, lack of rest.
- Fear of the repercussions of activity, which can lead to under-activity, physical deconditioning, isolation, boredom, introversion and depression.
- Loneliness, lack of social support and emotional stress.
- Stress from lack of finances leaving no safety net for survival needs (e.g., food, shelter)
- The hypervigilance loop - an *inner terrain* issue (see Chapter 15)
- Persistent undiagnosed infection and /or its autoimmune repercussions: **viral** e.g., Long-Covid 19, **chronic bacterial** (e.g., sinusitis), chlamydia pneumoniae, mycoplasma or **rickettsia** (such as Lyme disease or Ross River Fever).
- Gastrointestinal: **dysbiosis**, food intolerances and a poor diet. (See Chapters 8 and 9).
- Exposure to chemicals, molds, environmental pollution (an *external terrain* issue).
- Low vitamin D levels (may be particularly significant in fibromyalgia) or low vitamin B12. Recheck Vit D and B12 levels.

SWAT-like team for house/bedbound people

Currently 25% of people with ME/CFS are too unwell to travel to see their doctor or health professionals. It is also highly likely that COVID 19 will leave in its wake a massive increase in the numbers of people in this house or bedbound situation, potentially diagnosed with a long-COVID version of ME/CFS. Hence, I would like to see government funding for the formation of 'SWAT-like' teams of health professionals with expertise in ME/CFS who could make house calls in person or at the very least have online/virtual consultations with people with ME/CFS who are housebound or bedbound, including those in rural and regional areas, just as I was lucky enough to receive from Dr Lewis.

Having performed a thorough assessment, they could then liaise with local health professionals to educate and guide them as to how to best manage the person with ME/CFS, as is done with other chronic illnesses like diabetes. The effectiveness of this strategy could be evaluated.

FUTURE RESEARCH

"...medical students are taught that much of what they learn will be obsolete soon after they graduate."
SAMUEL ARBESMAN AUTHOR THE HALF LIFE OF FACTS.[1]

Research keeps bounding along, so much so that it is possible some of what I've shared here may be improved upon soon! Hence the need to keep abreast of what's happening. The websites I've included in the resources section will help you in this regard.

Once researchers develop a reliable diagnostic test for ME/CFS, it will not only confirm the diagnosis and validate the illness it will also allow more accurate assessment of treatment approaches. At this time, we may also be able to identify the subtype and severity of a person's ME/CFS, this would allow us to individually tailor and monitor the effectiveness or otherwise of different treatments over time.

Lifestyle Research - Where to Next?

The elephant in the room is this: why is there a general lack of funding for lifestyle research, like this eight-key program, that could be done now for ME/CFS or any other chronic illness? I believe there are for four main reasons.

- It's difficult to make a buck out of it. (Unlike medicines, supplements or surgery)
- Many people prefer easier solutions requiring less

commitment (like a pill). This might be reasonable if there was a pill.
- The double-blind trial, which became the gold standard in medical research 65 years ago, is not a methodology suited to holistic individualized lifestyle or mind-body research. Research into ME/CFS may benefit from new research methodologies, such as N of 1 (see Chapter 3).
- Since Pasteur's time the modern medical profession and medical research generally has underestimated how powerful people's self-healing capacities can be, believing lifestyle treatments to be 'wishy washy' and of minimal importance at best. The fields of epigenetics and neuroplasticity are shifting these monolithic beliefs.

In the meantime:
- In assessing a holistic program like the one presented in this book, we can utilize outcome measure study methods. When I say outcome measures, I am referring to symptoms like fatigue levels, sleep, headaches etc. and signs such as low blood pressure on prolonged standing (NMH or POTS) and other indirect tests like the NASA Lean Test *(See: A Doctor's Journey Back to Health Ch 3)* and inflammatory markers. Other outcome measurement tools include assessing activities of daily living (ADL's), ability to work and/or study, Quality of life measures and mental health questionnaires.
- Such an outcome research approach was employed by Dr George Jelinek and his colleagues when they assessed the effectiveness of their complete lifestyle program on Multiple Sclerosis with a five year follow up study.[2] A study to assess the effectiveness of the Micro-Rehab

approach suggested in this book on people with ME/CFS could use a similar methodology. For example, two similar groups of people (i.e., matched for age, sex etc.) with ME/CFS could be randomly assigned to either holistic paced rehab + usual medical care (i.e., the Treatment group) or just the usual medical care (the Control group). Those in the treatment group would receive an individually tailored program of holistic Micro-Rehab with inputs from appropriate experienced health professionals. Those in the control group would not be limited by the study parameters if they wished to explore other treatments but would only be assigned to usual medical care for the purposes of the study. Each group would log their progress.

- The above outcome-based trial could include an N=1 element in which each individual in the treatment group is encouraged to apply their own learnings, self-awareness and intuition to further individualize and tailor their program to meet their own unique situation.
- Long Covid rehab research, such as into box breathing, may be helpful for ME/CFS is worth keeping an eye on See: https://ne-np.facebook.com/MountSinaiNYC/videos/what-you-need-to-know-about-long-covid/333559008728400/
- Single lifestyle interventions I would like to see tested, on the grounds that they might encourage an epigenetic rejigging, include ice baths (Alastair Lynch found these helpful) and/or cold showers (see Chapter 12); Induced fever; Heat treatments; fasting; physical rehab elements (paced); mind-body techniques and a therapeutic three month trial of a low GI diet.

Other Promising Treatment Leads

- **Red Light therapy (Photobiomodulation)** is showing great promise in treating Parkinson's disease (PD). This treatment involves using red or near infrared light applied to the abdomen, which penetrates through the soft tissues much like a torch. How so? As a kid you may remember shining a torch through the palm of your hand and being delighted and a little surprised to see it shine all the way through. Research has shown a red light laser penetrates through the abdomen, through the colon and in so doing alters the microbiome. This change in the microbiome is thought to lead to a beneficial change in the chemicals released by these colonic bacteria which in turn improves the symptoms in Parkinson's disease.[3] Given so far it has been found to be safe it would be fascinating to see if it might help people with ME/CFS also.
- **Low dose Naltrexone (LDN)** - In terms of medications LDN is one which shows promise in small studies on people with Fibromyalgia thus far usually at a dose of 1 to 5 mg.[4-7] It is showing effectiveness in reducing pain and has an excellent safety profile. Just remember those with ME/CFS need to go low and slow (i.e., start at a lower dose of LDN and build slowly). Larger trials will be needed to confirm this (See ldnresearchtrust.org). No doubt other medications will be available soon to assist in managing symptoms, so keep informed.
- Nerve stimulation via a **Vagal nerve electric stimulator** placed on the neck has been shown to reduce inflammation and be helpful in Rheumatoid Arthritis and Inflammatory Bowel Disease. Trials for fibromyalgia are underway.[8,9]

- **Transcranial Magnetic Stimulation (TMS)** has shown promise in improving mood and chronic pain.[10]
- **Alterations** in the **gut microbiome** as a possible cause of ME/CFS may guide us towards treatments for ME/CFS like photobiomodulation, mentioned above, specific dietary interventions, probiotics etc. Watch this space.

As I shared with you in my introduction, while we would love to find a magic medicine or complementary therapy to do the hard work for us (and I'd be the first to cheer if it was found), we have yet to witness it. On the other hand, my personal experience with ME/CFS both as a patient and as a treating doctor has shown me that with patience and perseverance the 8 keys taught here can synergize together for you to travel your road in life with a renewed sense of well-being and enjoyment, where you are in the driver's seat not the disease.

Ruth, Tori and I wish you well on your journey.

APPENDIX 1

ME/CFS CANADIAN CLINICAL DIAGNOSTIC CRITERIA 2003 SUMMARY

To diagnose ME/CFS the patient must have the following:

- Pathological fatigue, post-exertional malaise, sleep problems, pain, two neurocognitive symptoms, and at least one symptom from two of the following categories: autonomic, neuroendocrine, immune.
- The fatigue and the other symptoms must persist, or be relapsing for at least six months in adults, or three months in children. A provisional diagnosis may be possible earlier.
- The symptoms cannot be explained by another illness.

Improved diagnostic accuracy can be obtained by measuring the severity and frequency of the listed symptoms**

Symptoms	Description of Symptoms
Pathological fatigue	A significant degree of new onset, unexplained, persistent or recurrent physical and/or mental fatigue that substantially reduces activity levels and which is not the result of ongoing exertion and not relieved by rest.
Post-exertional malaise	Mild exertion or even normal activities followed by malaise: the loss of physical and mental stamina and/or worsening of other symptoms. Recovery is delayed, taking more than 24 hours.
Sleep problems	Sleep is un-refreshing: disturbed quantity - daytime hypersomnia or night-time insomnia and/or disturbed rhythm – day/night reversal. Rarely is there no sleep problem.

Symptoms	Description of Symptoms
Pain	Pain is widespread, migratory or localized: Myalgia; arthralgia (without signs of inflammation); and/or headache - a new type, pattern or severity. Rarely is there no pain.
Two Neurocognitive symptoms	Impaired concentration, short term memory or word retrieval; hypersensitivity to light, noise or emotional overload; confusion; disorientation; slowness of thought; muscle weakness; ataxia.

At least one symptom from two of these categories:

Autonomic	Orthostatic intolerance: neurally mediated hypotension (NMH); postural orthostatic tachycardia (POTS); light headedness; extreme pallor; palpitations; exertional dyspnea; urinary frequency; irritable bowel syndrome (IBS); nausea.
Neuroendocrine	low body temperature; cold extremities; sweating; intolerance to heat or cold; reduced tolerance for stress; other symptoms worsen with stress; weight change; abnormal appetite.
Immune	recurrent flu-like symptoms; sore throats; tender lymph nodes; fevers; new sensitivities to food, medicines, odors or chemicals.

For doctors - Canadian Clinical Criteria Summary - http://sacfs.asn.au/download/consensus_overview_me_cfs.pdf (accessed March 2019)

http://www.me-de-patienten.nl/CCC Checklist.pdf (accessed March 2019)

ME/CFS Diagnostic Criteria National Academy of Sciences/Medicine 2015

The diagnosis requires that the unwell person have the following 3 symptoms:

1. FATIGUE – A substantial reduction or impairment in the ability to engage in pre-illness levels of occupational, educational, social, or personal activities, that persists for more than 6 months (3 months in children). The fatigue is often profound of new or definite onset (not lifelong), is not the result of ongoing excessive exertion, and is not substantially alleviated by rest.
2. Post Exertional Malaise (PEM)
3. Unrefreshing Sleep

One of the two following manifestations is also required:

1. Cognitive Impairment
2. Orthostatic Intolerance

NOTE: The diagnosis of ME/CFS should be questioned if people do not have these symptoms with moderate, substantial, or severe intensity for at least half of the time.

APPENDIX 2
SYMPTOM QUESTIONNAIRE

Name _____

Date filled in _____/_____/_____

Instructions: 1. Rank your symptoms in order of severity from 1 to 20 (1 being your most severe) in the left column. 2. Rate severity of symptoms by putting 0, 1, 2 or 3 beside each symptom ( )

Rank [ ]	Severity ( ) Absent (0); Mild (1); Moderate (2); Severe (3)	
[ ]	Post-exertional fatigue: loss of physical and mental stamina, fatigue made worse by physical exertion.	( )
[ ]	Long recovery period from exertion: takes more than 24 hours to recover to pre-exertion activity level.	( )
[ ]	Fatigue: persistent, marked fatigue that substantially reduces activity level.	( )
[ ]	Sleep disturbance: non-restorative sleep, insomnia, hypersomnia	( )
[ ]	Pain: in muscles, joints, headaches	( )
[ ]	Memory disturbance: poor short term memory.	( )
[ ]	Confusion and difficulty concentrating.	( )
[ ]	Difficulty retrieving words or saying the wrong word.	( )
[ ]	Gastrointestinal disturbance: diarrhoea, IBS.	( )
[ ]	Recurrent sore throat.	( )
[ ]	Recurrent flu-like symptoms.	( )
[ ]	Dizziness or weakness upon standing.	( )
[ ]	Change in body temperature, erratic body temperature, cold hands and feet.	( )
[ ]	Heat/cold intolerance.	( )
[ ]	Hot flushes, sweating episodes.	( )

[ ]	Marked weight change.	( )
[ ]	Breathless with exertion.	( )
[ ]	Tender lymph nodes: especially at sides of neck and under arms	( )
[ ]	Sensitive to light, noise, or odors.	( )
[ ]	Muscle weakness. New sensitivities to food/medications/chemicals.	( )
		Total Score ___

Other symptoms

_____

Aggravators

_____

_____

How good is your sleep on a scale of 1 to 5? (5 = good restorative sleep, 1 = no sleep) _____

How do you feel today on a scale of 1 to 10? (10 = terrific, 1 = totally bedridden) _____

_{Adapted from Myalgic Encephalomyelitis/Chronic Fatigue Syndrome: A Clinical Case Definition and Guidelines for Medical Practitioners. An Overview of the Canadian Consensus Document. Carruthers BM, van de Sande MI & inputs from ThinkGP (Part of Reed Exhibitions Australia Pty Ltd – ABN 47 000 142 921) Tower 2, 475 Victoria Avenue Chatswood NSW 2067}

APPENDIX 3

OTHER POSSIBLE CAUSES (DIFFERENTIAL DIAGNOSIS)

Conditions that may mimic or can coexist with CFS (alphabetically listed):

- Adrenal Insufficiency
- Anemia
- Cancer
- Celiac disease
- Chronic Viral infections e.g., EBV, CMV, hepatitis, HIV/AIDS, Long-COVID
- Craniocervical Instability/Atlantoaxial instability (More common in Ehler's Danlos Syndrome).
- Diabetes Mellitus
- Fibromyalgia
- Functional Neurological Disorder (FND)
- Hypothyroidism
- Heavy metal toxicity (proven by urine or hair analysis)
- Lyme Disease and other Rickettsial infections
- Multiple Sclerosis
- Obstructive Sleep Apnea (OSA)
- Orthostatic Hypotension
- Parkinson's disease (early)
- Polymyalgia Rheumatica
- Postural Orthostatic Tachycardia syndrome (POTS)
- Psychiatric disorders – anxiety depression, eating disorders (anorexia nervosa, blemia)
- Rheumatological diseases eg. Rheumatoid Arthritis, Lupus, Polymyalgia Rheumatica, Sjogren's Syndrome,

Marfans Syndrome, Ehlers Danlos Syndrome
- Sinoatrial node dysfunction leading to bradycardia (slow heart rate)
- Sleep Disorders – Sleep Apnoea, Restless Legs Syndrome
- Supplementation or medication side effect or interaction

These conditions may give you symptoms with similarities to CFS, including severe fatigue, and need to be excluded (see link below) by a thorough medical history, examination and medical testing.

https://emedicine.medscape.com/article/235980-differential

APPENDIX 4
WHOLE FOOD LOW GI DIET SUGGESTIONS

- Avoid sugar and high fructose corn syrup (called glucose syrup in Australia). Includes most confectionary bars, sweets and soft drinks. Replace sugar with rice syrup, stevia, small amounts of honey, evaporated coconut nectar, apple or pear juice concentrate (also in small amounts) or a combination of these. Stevia is particularly good as it is zero GI.
- Eat lots of vegetables of a variety of colors and some fresh fruit each day (organic or spray free if possible).
- Avoid dairy milk and confine dairy products to cultured versions e.g., yoghurt, kefir, parmesan cheese, you could try lactose free cheeses too. White cheeses may also be better tolerated than cheddars.
- Include a smallish serving of a high protein food **every** time you eat/snack (see below), e.g., Fish (tins OK), nuts, nut butters, seeds, chicken, lean red meat, beans, tofu, tempeh, cheese, plain yoghurt, soy milk, eggs, protein powders, biscuits or cakes made with almond meal but no sugar.
- Forego refined grain products e.g., white rice and white flour products (bread, cakes, biscuits etc.) Substitute with small serves of wholemeal products and grains, e.g., brown rice, quinoa, almond meal products, wholemeal flour.
- Use healthier oils such as cold pressed olive oil and avocados. Avoid margarine and deep-fried food as

a priority, as these foods tend to contain trans-fats. Although **trans fats** are edible, consuming trans fats has been shown to increase the risk of coronary artery disease in part by raising levels of low-density lipoprotein (LDL, often termed "bad cholesterol"), lowering levels of high-density lipoprotein (HDL, often termed "good cholesterol"), increasing triglycerides in the bloodstream and **promoting systemic inflammation** https://www.ncbi.nlm.nih.gov/pmc/articles/PMC5986484/

- Try a Chia Pod or make your own – soak overnight in fridge 25g of chia seeds in half to two thirds of a cup of water. In morning add yoghurt and chopped up or stewed fruit e.g., Mango, apples + cinnamon +/- honey. Chia seeds are a good source of fibre and nutrition, including protein, calcium and omega 3 oils, avoid heating them beyond warm, as this maintains the quality of the delicate good fats contained within the seeds. Chia seeds help with collagen production in our bodies. So, sit back and watch your nails grow stronger!
- Add cultured foods (stored in your fridge), such as sauerkraut, kombucha, kimchee, kefir, or yoghurt to your daily routine foods.
- Bone broth can also be very nurturing and nutritious, try it as a chicken soup made with the drumsticks, good recipes are available on Dr Google! There are also dehydrated versions you can purchase (ask a health food shop) and add to soups or casseroles.
- Dark chocolate (70% to 85% cocoa) can improve energy levels and can be a healthy dietary dessert. See Which Chocolate is Best for Your Heart? – Cleveland Clinic

Extra Protein Snack Tips
(www.betterhealth.vic.gov.au/healt/healthyliving/protein)

- Try a peanut butter (or other nutbutter e.g., almond butter) sandwich. Remember to use natural peanut butter (or any other nut paste) with no added salt, sugar or other fillers.
- Low-fat cottage or ricotta cheese is high in protein and can go in your scrambled eggs, casserole, mashed potato or pasta dish. Or spread it on your toast in the morning.
- Nuts and seeds are fantastic in salads, with vegetables and served on top of curries. Try toasting some pine nuts or flaked almonds and putting them in your green salad.
- Beans are great in soups, casseroles, and pasta sauces. Try tipping a drained can of cannellini beans into your favourite vegetable soup recipe or casserole.
- A plate of hummus and freshly cut vegetable sticks as a snack or hummus spread on your sandwich will give you easy extra protein at lunchtime.
- Greek yoghurt is a protein rich food that you can use throughout the day. Add some on your favourite breakfast cereal, put a spoonful on top of a bowl of pumpkin soup or serve it as dessert with some fresh fruit.
- Eggs are a versatile and easy option that can be enjoyed on their own or mixed in a variety of dishes.

APPENDIX 5
BELLY BREATHING

Background

Our breathing pattern can not only reflect our state of mind but can make our ME/CFS symptoms better or worse. When we are anxious or stressed we tend to breathe more quickly and shallowly, into our upper chest. This lowers the C02 in our blood stream and this can worsen our symptoms. In contrast when we breathe more deeply into our belly, more air moves into the lower part of our lungs. This happens because the diaphragm, the sheet of curved muscle that divides the chest from the abdomen, flattens out.

When it flattens, it triggers a relaxation response via a nerve pathway (a two-way parasympathetic wiring system if you like) called the vagus nerve. This signals chemicals to be released into our nervous system that instantly help us to de-stress and relax.

So, taking two or three slow, deep breaths is a bit like self-medicating without the medication. It can take a bit of practice to learn, so don't be too fussed about getting it perfect straight away. It will become easier with practice.

Practice

1. Slow Belly Breathing

Place one hand on your belly and your other hand on your chest. Now just notice the pattern of your breathing....There is no right or wrong here, you are simply noticing the pattern of your breathing. Are both hands moving? ...Is one hand moving more than the other? Just notice the pattern.

Now leaving one hand on your belly, rest your other hand. Now breathe out naturally and fully. ....As you breathe in, see if you can breathe slowly down into your belly. ...Try that again, breathing out fully first. .. then breathing in slowly into your belly.

If this is difficult, try again, only this time, without moving your head, look upwards with your eyes. Breathe out fully...and then breathe in slowly into your belly. Looking upwards with your eyes while practicing, can help you to learn how to breathe more deeply, as it will cause you to do so automatically. Once you get the idea you won't need to look up any more, except maybe to help you at very stressful times. You might also like to give a sigh as you breathe out to further release tension.

Timing

I suggest you take 3 slow deep box breaths regularly throughout the day, at least 3 to 5 times. This will help you to unwind so that by days end you will feel more relaxed and more able to sleep.

Triggers

Are there any triggers during the day that could remind you to do this?

For example, anytime you find yourself waiting - like on the phone, for your computer to reboot, in a queue, on the loo or at a red light. Before or after meals is a good idea too, as stimulating the vagus nerve can aid digestion. Think of triggers that would work for you and place sticky dots or notes in spots you tend to frequent during the day so that when you see these sticky reminders you breathe slow and low for at least three in and out breath cycles.

2. Box Breathing

This technique slows down your breathing rate thus increasing CO_2 in the bloodstream and reducing hyperventilation (over breathing).

It reduces anxiety and has been beneficial for both long Covid1 and ME/CFS.

Step 1: Breathe out naturally, then breathe out further to gently empty your lungs without forcing.

Step 2: Breathe in counting to three or four slowly, whatever is most comfortable. Feel the air enter your lungs, saying, "In, two, three, (four)".

Step 3: Hold your breath for 3 to 4 seconds. "Hold, two, three, (four)." Try to avoid inhaling or exhaling during this time.

Step 4: Slowly exhale through your mouth. "Out, two, three, (four)".

Step 5: Breathe in and complete the box shape with even sides, "In, two, three, (four)".

Repeat steps 1 to 4 until you feel re-centred.

3. Sleep Aid

If you are having trouble sleeping, try this in bed. Place one hand on your belly and focus on slow belly breaths until you drift off to sleep. Your belly should rise and fall with the breath under your hand.

https://ne-np.facebook.com/MountSinaiNYC/videos/what-you-need-to-know-about-long-covid/333559008728400/

APPENDIX 6

MEDITATION AND RELAXATION EXERCISES

Guidelines for practice

These three restoring exercises are best practiced at least once or twice a day with your body placed in a balanced and symmetrical position either sitting or lying down. You or someone close to you may wish to make a recording of the instructions (speak at a slow, easy pace) to playback. Alternatively you can purchase an audio recording I've made (Restoring Balance) at my website www.drstevensommer.com.

Sitting upright in a basic kitchen chair is ideal, but if this is too difficult, try lying down on supportive ground with a flat pillow for your head, knees bent if need be. The idea here is to be slightly uncomfortable so you stay awake during the exercise. If this is not possible then by all means try out different positions and see what works best for you.

An extra layer like a shawl or a jumper might be needed. The second exercise, the muscle relaxation, can also be practiced in bed at night to help you to fall asleep. In this situation, follow the instructions initially and then as you drift off, let the sleep train carry you away rather than keep following.

Other general guidelines include practicing before food rather than after, and you might even consider a gentle stretch for your body before you start. So before breakfast and before dinner are good times. It might mean waking up 10 minutes earlier, starting out your day on a clear note, then leaving behind the day's events by meditating before dinner. If this is not possible then any time is better than missing out. The key here is **timetabling** it as a priority time just for you. Other members of your household may need to be told that you are off limits during your restoring breaks…and leave the phone off or to take care of itself.

Senses Awareness Meditation (5 – 10 Minutes)

Start this exercise sitting upright in a chair, your feet resting flat on the floor and your back straight. Keep your head upright as well so that its balanced, taking any pressure off your neck muscles.

Now, gently close your eyes and take two slow deep breaths letting the chair take your body's weight completely as you breath out.   {Pause}

. ...Maybe take one more of those deep breaths and if you like, give a sigh as you breathe out, sighing away any tension. (Repeat this if it feels good to do)

Good.

Now become aware of your feet where they touch the floor. Wriggle your toes if this helps; then rest them.... {Pause}

Become aware of the weight of your body in the chair. ...Feel where the chair is pressing against your buttocks and your back....{Pause}

Perhaps you can become aware of the clothes where they touch the skin. .. {Pause}

See if you can feel the play of air on your face and your hands...{Pause}

Let any sense of smell come into your awareness as you breathe in through your nose...{Pause}

Allow any tastes present in your mouth to be detected...{Pause}

Now shift your attention to listening. Take in all the sounds you can hear both near and far, moving from one sound to the next...... {lengthy Pause at least 2 minutes}

If you become aware your mind is focusing on other things, like thoughts or feelings, not to worry, just let them be and whenever you are able, return your attention to simply listening.... {Pause}

Let the listening stretch right out into the distance...{lengthy Pause}

Good...good.

Now take another slow deep breath, returning your attention to the feeling of the weight of your body sitting in the chair. {Pause}

Wriggle your toes and your fingers and just in your own time when you're ready, gently open your eyes.

Soften & Flow Meditation (10- 20 minutes) for easing emotional & physical tension

Once again find a balanced position either sitting upright in a chair, or you can lie on your back on a firm-ish surface with a pillow beneath your head; body straight; legs either resting straight or bent at the knees.

Now, gently close your eyes. Let's start by taking 2 slow rich breaths, letting the air flow out fully with each breath. **[pause]**

Maybe take one more of those deep breaths, letting the chair or the floor take your body's weight completely as you breathe out.

Good. Now we are going to scan our body, becoming aware of any areas where we might be holding tension. Just observing these areas noting any physical or emotional tension, without the need to change them, just acknowledging what's there.

So let's start with our legs. Observe your feet….Are your feet holding any tension?…What about your calves?….or your thighs? How do they feel?

Now shift your awareness to your buttocks….Acknowledge if there is any tension there. **[pause]** Now to your back? **[pause]** Your shoulders?… **[pause]** Your neck?… **[pause]** Your head? …. **[pause]** Your face? **[pause]**

Become aware if any tensions are held in your chest….what about your abdomen **[pause]**. It is common to find emotional tension held in our belly or chest areas; perhaps tune into these areas again….

Now choose one area that you have found where you might be holding some emotional or physical tension. Observe it again....acknowledge it.

Now gently breathe into it, and as you breathe out say in your mind - "soften and flow....soften and flow"....Continue to gently breathe into it and every now and again as you breathe out say, "soften and flow, soften and flow."

[BIG pause]

Acknowledge it again. Sit with it if you like. There is no need to resist it, just be with it, breathe into it and .... "soften and flow, soften and flow."

[BIG pause]

If you find your mind wandering, not to worry, just as often as you are able, bring it gently back to the area of observation and .... "soften and flow....soften and flow."

[BIG pause]

You might find the tension is easing off a little now and you might wish to choose another area to relieve of tension or might like to just continue to rest quietly.

[brief pause]

Otherwise, if you're ready to complete, just begin to deepen your breath a little. Wriggle your toes and your fingers. And in your own time when you're ready, open your eyes.

YOGA Nidra Deep Muscle Relaxation (15-30 minutes)

Spend some time now tuning into and relaxing your body. Find a balanced position lying on your back on the floor with a pillow beneath your head; body straight; or you could sit upright in a chair. If you are using this as an aid for sleeping then lying on your back in your bed ready for sleep is fine.

Now, gently close your eyes. Begin by taking two slow, deep breaths. Breathing in as fully as is comfortable and letting the air flow out fully each time, giving a sigh as you breathe out if you like.

…… Now allow your breathing to return to its own natural rhythm. Become aware of your whole body. Feel your body's weight. You might like to adjust your position, so that it feels balanced and comfortable… Take another slow deep breath, allowing the surface you are lying on to take your weight completely….

Now clearly picture your feet in your mind, wriggle your toes if it helps and let your feet relax…, soften…, loosen…, allowing a deep relaxation to flow into your feet…..{Pause}

Turn your attention to your calves, notice how they feel, is one calf tighter than the other? … Just observe how your calves feel without the need for judgment or comment and allow the calves to relax… Let the relaxation flow deeply through the muscles of the calves…softening…,loosening…, releasing…{Pause}

Turn your attention now to your thighs. Notice how they feel… feel the back of your thighs… feel the front of your thighs… allow them to release, let go… Allow your thighs to relax…, soften…, loosen… {Pause}

Bring your attention now to your buttocks… How do they feel?… Allow the muscles to relax… Letting go of any tension, let the tension flow out, down your legs and out through the tips of your toes…. {Pause}

Focus now on your belly… Notice how it feels …, allow it to soften… Feel a relaxation spreading around from your belly to your lower back…… Feel the relaxation spreading right through, calm and ease…..ease and calm…{Pause}

Shift your attention now to your chest, notice how it moves with your breath.., as you breathe with your own natural rhythm.... Feel the chest wall soften..., loosen..., all the way around to your back...{Pause}

Become aware of your arms. Feel the weight of your arms; relaxing your upper arms; your elbows; your forearms; your wrists and your hands...{Pause}

Bring your attention to your shoulders. Shrug them if it helps... Notice how they feel... Imagine any tension flowing down through your arms and out through the tips of your fingers. Allow your shoulders to hang loose..., soften,.. release...

...{Pause}

Become aware of your neck... Feel your muscles soften..., relax..., release...

...{Pause}

Allow the jaw to hang loose..., the lips to part slightly..., relaxing the mouth..., your cheeks.. softening and releasing...... Feel your eyes relax.... your forehead smooth over..... Feel the top of your head loosening and releasing ...., the sides of your head... the back of your head......{Pause}

Rest with your body's weight.... ...{Pause}

Now let's take a further mental inventory of the body, deepening our relaxation as we send a message to let go and relax: To the toes of the feet... soles..,heels...,back of the feet......{Pause}

Sending a message to let go and relax to the:

ankles.., calves..., shins.... and your knees......{Pause}

Sending a message to let go and relax to the:

Back of the knees.., thighs..., back of the thighs.... and your buttocks......{Pause}

APPENDIX 6 MEDITATION AND RELAXATION EXERCISES

Sending a message to let go and relax to the:

Lower back.., middle back…, upper back…. and your shoulders…… {Pause}

Sending a message to let go and relax:

To the upper arms.., elbows…, forearms…. and wrists…… {Pause}

Sending a message to let go and relax:

To the palm of the hands.., back of the hands…, fingers …. and your thumbs. …{Pause}

Sending a message to let go and relax:

To the belly.., chest…,neck…. and your jaw… …{Pause}

Sending a message to let go and relax:

To your mouth.., nose…, cheeks…. and your eyes… …{Pause}

Sending a message to let go and relax:

To your eyelids.., eyebrows…, forehead…. and your ears… …{Pause}

Sending a message to let go and relax:

To your temples.., top of your head…, sides of your head …. and the back of the head……{Pause}

Feeling waves of relaxation now, flowing through your entire body as you simply let go and relax…{Pause} Resting with the ease of it all…. the ease of it all.

{BIG PAUSE - at least five minutes}

Feeling the weight of your body and the ease of it all…the ease of it all.

{BIG PAUSE until ready to complete}

{Softly spoken} Now gently deepen your breath….{Pause}… wriggle the toes a little…. and your fingers … and just in your own time.., when you're ready.., gently open your eyes.

FURTHER READING

Germer C. The Mindful Path to Self-Compassion. Guilford 2009 New York.

Neff K, Self Compassion. Hodder and Stoughton 2011.

Thich Nhat Hanh. The Miracle of Mindfulness 1975.

Gawler I, Bedson P. Meditation an In-Depth Guide. Allen & Unwin 2010, Sydney Australia.

Kabat-Zinn. Wherever You Are There You Are. Hyperion 2011. New York.

Kornfield J. A Path of Heart. Bantam Doubleday Publishing Group Dec 1993 USA.

Salzberg S. Real Happiness: The Power of Meditation: A 28-Day Program Kindle Edition with Audio/Video workman Publishing 2010 and 2020 (2nd ed).

APPENDIX 7

AUTOMATIC NEGATIVE THOUGHTS (ANTS) AND POSITIVE EMOTIONAL THOUGHTS (PETS)

Automatic Negative Thoughts (ANTS)

(these can occur consciously and subconsciously)

ANTICIPATION OF SYMPTOMS

Egs   Oh no! I've over done it again!. – Now I have to recover again.

I'm going to feel unwell for days.

If I do this, I'll feel exhausted.

I won't have enough energy to go out tonight.

ATTENTION ON SYMPTOMS

Egs   My legs are hurting again.

I feel so tired.

The fatigue and pain are so hard to bear.

I can't live a normal life with this pain.

What's this new pain?

BODY SCANNING

Egs   How painful are my legs, my head? How's my stomach feel? etc

WILL I EVER GET BETER?

Egs   What if I never get better?

Nothing seems to help.

I'll never get better.

FRUSTRATION & ANGER AT BEING ILL

Egs
I'm sick of feeling sick!

I wish these symptoms would just go away!

I can't stand this anymore!

NOBODY UNDERSTANDS ME

Egs
People are judging me, they think there's nothing wrong with me.

I wish they could experience what I do just for a week!

I'm all alone with this.

When I'm feeling so awful and in pain some people say to me:

"You look so great" or "Good to see you better at last." or "Are you still sick!!??" or "What's wrong with you, you look okay!!?"

DIETARY WORRIES

Egs
I ate the wrong thing, now I'll suffer for it.

I can't eat that. I must stick to my diet.

SLEEP WORRIES

Egs
I can't sleep, I'm going to feel terrible tomorrow.

If only I could have a decent sleep.

I'm awake again, now I'll never get back to sleep and I'll pay for it.

OTHER

I feel I am a burden to my family, especially my partner.

APPENDIX 7

Positive Emotional Thoughts (PETS) (Recall one person's PET can be another person's ANT, so only apply those that make *you feel* relieved - add your own to those below.)

ANTICIPATION OF IMPROVEMENT

Egs
I'm on the road to recovery from CFS.
I have bounced back before – so I can do it again!
You can do it!
Remember how tough you are.
It doesn't matter – there is time. "I'm a tough mother!"
New treatments are being discovered all the time.
Look how far I've come.

SYMPTOM REASSURANCE

Egs
It's OK. It's not an emergency.
I've experienced this before and recovered.
I can't sleep, not to worry, I'll meditate or read instead.

REFRAMING

Egs
It's OK I'm doing anxiety right now.
It's OK I'm doing pain right now

BODY SCANNING

Eg
Listen to my body
No need to be anxious for I'm listening to you now.
Soften and Flow meditation
I'm home again my darling body so you can relax.

BIG PICTURE

Egs
I don't have to solve it all today.
Tomorrow is another day.

This too will pass.

New research is happening all the time.

DO SOMETHING
Egs

It's OK to ask for help.

It's OK to express my needs.

It's OK to express my emotions

It's OK to cry.

Breathe – relax.

Battery charge (meditate)

Move!

Stroll in nature

Sit in nature/Be in nature

Think happy – smile.

Do something I like – read, watch movie, sit in my garden, go to a park, or beach, listen to music, talk to loved one.

Pain equals heat pack or cold pack

LETTING IT GO
Egs

Pace, rest, enjoy life.

Let go and let God.

Pray.

Ask for help.

TUNING IN
Egs

I'll have a 'Nanna Nap' as soon as I can.

I'll rest now.

I need to move.

Pace (remember the rest/activity dance)

I need to talk about this.

APPENDIX 7

PEP TALK

Egs — Don't take people's comments to heart – smile and reply: "thank you." – "I'm getting there." – "I'm improving gradually."

Look in the mirror every day and say: "You're marvelous to be surviving; you have achieved so much to get to this point; I'm okay as I am; I don't have to please anyone."

We're working on it.

If Plan A doesn't work, we'll find a Plan B (C or D etc.)

I am special and I am loved.

GRATITUDE

Recall three positive experiences from the day, each night before bed (Egs -a laugh, a bird's song, a thing of beauty).

Savor what I do have.

Before you eat, pause.

FURTHER RESOURCES

Websites

www.emerge.org.au

https://mecfs.org.au/

http://www.cfidsselfhelp.org/

http://www.meassociation.org.uk/

Visit ME/CFS sites:

(Accessed December 2020)

Australia (Accessed December 2020)

USA (Accessed December 2020)

UK (Accessed December 2020)

Other Links

www.drstevensommer.com

https://drdaniellewis.com.au/ (Accessed July 2021)

https://www.healthrising.org/ (Accessed December 2020)

https://phoenixrising.me/ (Accessed December 2020)

https://www.betterhealth.vic.gov.au/health/conditionsandtreatments/chronic-fatigue-syndrome-cfs (Accessed December 2020)

https://www.sbs.com.au/ondemand/video/1334946883764/insight-chronic-fatigue-syndrome (Accessed December 2020)

https://ne-np.facebook.com/MountSinaiNYC/videos/what-you-need-to-know-about-long-covid/333559008728400/

Fact Sheets

https://emerge.org.au/category/about-mecfs/fact-sheets/#.Xdo4BtVS8dc

Includes fact sheets on diagnosis, management, pacing, research and explanations for family and friends.

Books

Barton A. Recovery from CFS – 50 personal stories. Author House UK Ltd 2008.

McIntyre A. Chronic Fatigue Syndrome – a practical guide. Thorsons London 1998:1-33.

Vallings R. The Pocket Guide to Chronic Fatigue Syndrome ME – Key Facts and Tips for Improved Health. Calico Publishing 2017, Auckland.

Vallings R. Chronic Fatigue Syndrome ME - Symptom, Diagnosis, Management. Calico Publishing 2012, Auckland.

Campbell B. The Patient's Guide to Chronic Fatigue Syndrome and Fibromyalgia. 2011 Available at: http://www.cfidsselfhelp.org/library/the-patients-guide-chronic-fatigue-syndromefibromyalgia

Lynch A, Blucher P. Taking Nothing For Granted. A sportsman's fight against Chronic Fatigue. Harper Collins 2005. eBook available from Harper.

Sommer SJ. Finding Hope - when facing serious disease. Inspiring Stories, Healing Insights and Health Research. Amazon.com 2017. Also available from drstevensommer.com

Marchant J. Cure. Text publishing Melbourne 2016.

FURTHER RESOURCES

Look up ME/CFS Clinics in your local area or nearest city like:

https://drdaniellewis.com.au/ (Accessed July 2021)

http://www.austin.org.au/Adult_CFS (Accessed August 2020)

https://www.epworth.org.au/Our-Services/rehabilitation/Pages/chronic-fatigue-program.aspx (Accessed August 2020)

https://www.alfredhealth.org.au/services/chronic-fatigue-clinic (Accessed August 2020)

https://www.statnews.com/2017/09/25/chronic-fatigue-syndrome-cdc/

https://activehealthclinic.com.au Nathan Butler (Accessed July 2021)

https://www.medpagetoday.com/rheumatology/generalrheumatology/78944.

REFERENCES ME/CFS

Introduction

1. Sommer SJ. *A Doctor's Journey Back to Health* www.drstevensommer.com *2021*
2. ME/CFS The biomedical basis, diagnosis, treatment and management. International Research Symposium Geelong Australia, March 12-15.
3. https://www.newscientist.com/article/2121162-metabolic-switch-may-bring-on-chronic-fatigue-syndrome/
4. https://www.medpagetoday.com/rheumatology/generalrheumatology/78944
5. Lillie EO, Patay B, Diamant J, et al. The n-of-1 clinical trial: the ultimate strategy for individualizing medicine? Per Med. 2011 Mar; 8(2): 161–173.
6. https://www.mcri.edu.au/news/researchers-discover-two-treatments-induce-peanut-allergy-remission-children
7. https://www.theguardian.com/society/2021/dec/02/people-microdosing-on-psychedelics-to-improve-wellbeing-during-pandemic
8. pdwarrior.com
9. Hadgkiss EJ, Jelinek GA, Weiland TJ et al. Health-related quality of life outcomes at 1 and 5 years after a residential retreat promoting lifestyle modification for people with multiple sclerosis, Neurol Sci. 2013 Feb;34(2):187-95.
10. Uhrbrand A, Stenager E , Pedersen MS et al. Parkinson's disease and intensive exercise therapy--a systematic review and meta-analysis of randomized controlled trials Review J Neurol Sci 2015;353(1-2):9-19.
11. https://www.nobelprize.org/prizes/medicine/2000/summary/
12. Doidge N. The Brain That Changes Itself: Stories of Personal Triumph from the Frontiers of Brain Science. Viking Press 2007.

Chapter 1 Ruth's Story circa 2008

1. Gador R. An Unexpected Friendship. Emerge Summer 2013, Vol 32 No (4): 18.

Chapter 2 Changing the Terrain - The Power of Lifestyle

1. https://www.journals.uchicago.edu/doi/abs/10.1086/649300?journalCode=osiris
2. Cohen, I. Bernard, "Foreword", in the Dover edition (1957) of: Bernard, Claude, *An Introduction to the Study of Experimental Medicine* (originally published in 1865; first English translation by Henry Copley Greene, published by Macmillan & Co., Ltd., 1927).
3. Cannon, Walter B, The Wisdom of the Body. New York: Norton 1932.
4. https://www.ncbi.nlm.nih.gov/pmc/articles/PMC7266578/
5. https://www.theguardian.com/world/2020/aug/26/obesity-increases-risk-of-covid-19-death-by-48-study-finds
6. Ulrich R S. View through a Window May Influence Recovery from Surgery. Science 1984;224 (4647): 420-1.
7. Beauchemin KM, Hays P. Dying in the dark: sunshine, gender and outcomes in myocardial infarction. J R Soc Med 1998;91:352–354.

8. Beauchemin KM, Hays P Sunny hospital rooms expedite recovery from severe and refractory depressions. J Affect Disord 1996 Sep 9;40(1-2):49-51.
9. Ornish D, Brown SE, Scherwitz L W et al. Can lifestyle changes reverse coronary heart disease? Lancet 1990:336: 129-133.
10. Ornish D. Dr Dean Ornish 's program for reversing heart disease. New York: Random House, 1990.
11. Moyers B. Healing and the Mind. Doubleday New York 1993:87-113.
12. News. US insurance company covers lifestyle therapy. Br Med J 1993;307:465.
13. Ibid 1., p79-94.
14. Ornish D, Weidner G,Fair WR et al. Intensive lifestyle changes may affect progression of prostate cancer, the Journal of Urology September 2005; Vol. 174, 1065–1070.
15. Ibid 1., p95-107.
16. Frattaroli J, Weidner G, Dnistrian AM, et al. Clinical events in prostate cancer lifestyle trial: results from two years of follow-up. Urology. 2008 Dec;72(6):1319-23.
17. Ornish D, Magbanua MJ, Weidner G et al. Changes in prostate gene expression in men undergoing an intensive nutrition and lifestyle intervention. Proc Natl Acad Sci U S A. 2008 Jun 17;105(24):8369-74.
18. Ornish D, Lin J, Chan JM et al. Effect of comprehensive lifestyle changes on telomerase activity and telomere length in men with biopsy-proven low-risk prostate cancer: 5-year follow-up of a descriptive pilot study, Lancet Oncol. 2013 Oct;14(11):1112-20.
19. Jellinek G. Taking Control of Multiple Sclerosis -- Natural and Medical Therapies to Prevent its Progression. Melbourne: Hyland House Publishing 2005.
20. Esparza ML, Sasaki S, Kesteloot H. Nutrition, latitude and Multiple Sclerosis mortality: an ecologic study. Am J Epidemiol 1995;142:733-7.
21. Swank RL, Dugan BB. Effect of low saturated fat diet in early and late cases of Multiple Sclerosis. Lancet 1990;336:37-9.
22. Swank RL. Multiple Sclerosis: fat-oil relationship Nutrition 1991;7:368-76.
23. Hadgkiss EJ, Jelinek GA, Weiland TJ et al. Health-related quality of life outcomes at 1 and 5 years after a residential retreat promoting lifestyle modification for people with multiple sclerosis, Neurol Sci. 2013 Feb;34(2):187-95.
24. Uhrbrand A, Stenager E , Pedersen MS et al. Parkinson's disease and intensive exercise therapy--a systematic review and meta-analysis of randomized controlled trials Review J Neurol Sci 2015;353(1-2):9-19.
25. https://www.acpm.org/page/lmresearch (accessed May 2019)
26. Jackson R1, Lawes CM, Bennett DA, et al. Treatment with drugs to lower blood pressure and blood cholesterol based on an individual's absolute cardiovascular risk. Lancet. 2005 Jan 29-Feb 4;365(9457):434-41.
27. https://www.cdc.gov/cancer/lung/basic_info/risk_factors.htm
28. https://www.asbestos.com/asbestos/smoking/
29. Lillie EO, Patay B, Diamant J, et al. The n-of-1 clinical trial: the ultimate strategy for individualizing medicine? Per Med. 2011 Mar; 8(2): 161–173.

Chapter 3 Finding Hope - A Treatment Plan

1. *Sommer SJ. Finding Hope - when facing serious disease. Inspiring Stories, Healing Insights and Health Research. Amazon.com 2017. Also available from* www.drstevensommer.com
2. Lynch A, Blucher P. Taking Nothing For Granted. A sportsman's fight against Chronic Fatigue. Harper Collins 2005. E6:11. EBook available from Harper.

3. Lillie EO, Patay B, Diamant J, et al. The n-of-1 clinical trial: the ultimate strategy for individualizing medicine? Per Med. 2011 Mar; 8(2): 161–173.
4. Barton A. Recovery from CFS – 50 personal stories. Author House UK Ltd 2008.
5. Jason L, Torres-Harding S, Njok M. The face of CFS in the U.S. CFIDS Chronicle 2006;16–21. http://www.researchgate.net/profile/Leonard_Jason/publication/236995875.
6. Solomon L, Reeves WC. Factors influencing the diagnosis of chronic fatigue syndrome. Arch Int Med 2004;164(20):2241–5.
7. Pajediene E, Bileviciute-Ljungar I, Friberg D. Sleep patterns among patients with chronic fatigue: A polysomnography-based study. Clin Respir J. 2018 Apr;12(4):1389-1397.
8. Bested AC, Marshall LM. Review of Myalgic Encephalomyelitis/Chronic Fatigue Syndrome: an evidence-based approach to diagnosis and management by clinicians. Rev Environ Health. 2015;30(4):237. doi: 10.1515/reveh-2015-0026.
9. Ocon A J, Messer Z R, Medow M S, et al. Increasing orthostatic stress impairs neurocognitive functioning in chronic fatigue syndrome with postural tachycardia syndrome. Clin Sci (Lond). 2012; 122: 227-238.
10. Bateman L, Bested A C, Bonilla HF, et al. Myalgic Encephalomyelitis/Chronic Fatigue Syndrome: Essentials of Diagnosis and Management. Mayo Clinic Proceedings Consensus Recommendations. Open Access August 25, 2021.
11. DOI:https//doi.org/10.1016/j.mayocp.2021.07.004   see link: Read it here

Chapter 4 Integrating Complementary Therapies

1. Porter NS, Jason LA, Boulton A, et al. *Alternative medical interventions used in the treatment and management of myalgic encephalomyelitis/chronic fatigue syndrome and fibromyalgia.* J Altern Complement Med. *2010 Mar;16(3):235-49.*
2. https://www.ncbi.nlm.nih.gov/pmc/articles/PMC4740396/
3. Biedermann L, Rogler G. The intestinal microbiota: its role in health and disease. Eur J Pediatr. 2015 Feb;174(2):151-67.
4. Brandt LJ. Fecal Microbiota Transplant: Respice, Adspice, Prospice. J Clin Gastroenterol. 2015 Nov-Dec;49 Suppl 1:S65-8.
5. Borody TJ, Nowak A, Torres M, et al. Bacteriotherapy in chronic fatigue syndrome: a retrospective review. Am J Gastroenterol. 2012;107(suppl 1):S591–S592.
6. Nathan N. On Hope and Healing: For those who have fallen through the medical cracks. Et Alia Press, Arkansas 2010:23-38.
7. Maric D, Brkic S, Tomic S et al. Multivitamin mineral supplementation in patients with chronic fatigue syndrome. Med Sci Monit. 2014 Jan 14;20:47-53.
8. Berkovitz S, Ambler G, Jenkins M, Thurgood S. Serum 25-hydroxy vitamin D levels in chronic fatigue syndrome: a retrospective survey. Int J Vitam Nutr Res 2009;79(4):250–4.
9. Bradley R, Schloss J, Brown D, et al. The effects of Vitamin D on acute viral respiratory infections: a rapid review Adv Integr Med 2020 Aug 3. doi: 10.1016/j.aimed.2020.07.011. Online ahead of print.
10. Entrenas M, Luis C, Entrenas M, et al. Effect of calcifediol treatment and best available therapy versus best available therapy on intensive care unit admission and mortality among patients hospitalized for COVID-19: A pilot randomized clinical study. The Journal of Steroid Biochemistry and Molecular Biology Volume 203, October 2020, 105751.

11. Regland B, Andersson M, Abrahamsson L, Bagby J, Dyrehag LE, et al. Increased concentrations of homocysteine in the cerebrospinal fluid in patients with fibromyalgia and chronic fatigue syndrome. Scand J Rheumatol 1997;26(4):301–7.
12. Bested AC, Marshall LM. Review of Myalgic Encephalomyelitis/Chronic Fatigue Syndrome: an evidence-based approach to diagnosis and management by clinicians. Rev Environ Health. 2015;30(4):243.
13. Regland B, Forsmark S, Halaouate L, et al. Response to vitamin B12 and folic acid in myalgic encephalomyelitis and fibromyalgia. PLoS One. 2015 Apr 22;10(4):e0124648.
14. Haoyang Lu, Xinzhou Liu, Yulin Deng et al. DNA methylation, a hand behind neurodegenerative diseases. Front Aging Neurosci. 2013; 5: 85.
15. https://www.youtube.com/watch?v=_akIWiUIjoU *(accessed October 2020)*
16. Cortese C, Motti C. MTHFR gene polymorphism, homocysteine and cardiovascular disease. Public Health Nutr. 2001 Apr;4(2B):493-7.
17. Kirsch SH, Herrmann W, Kruse V, et al. One year B-vitamins increases serum and whole blood folate forms and lowers plasma homocysteine in older Germans. Clin Chem Lab Med. 2015 Feb;53(3):445-52.
18. Keser I, Ilich JZ, Vrkić N, et al. Folic acid and vitamin B(12) supplementation lowers plasma homocysteine but has no effect on serum bone turnover markers in elderly women: a randomized, double-blind, placebo-controlled trial. Nutr Res. 2013 Mar;33(3):211-9.
19. Li C, Wu X, Liu S, et al. Role of Resolvins in the Inflammatory Resolution of Neurological Diseases. Front Pharmacol. 2020 May 8;11:612. doi: 10.3389/fphar.2020.00612. eCollection 2020. PMID: 32457616 Free PMC article.
20. Puri BK. The use of eicosapentaenoic acid in the treatment of chronic fatigue syndrome. Prostaglandins Leukot Essent Fatty Acids 2004;70(4):399–401.
21. Puri BK. Long-chain polyunsaturated fatty acids and the pathophysiology of myalgic encephalomyelitis (chronic fatigue syndrome). J Clin Pathol 2007;60:122–4.
22. Prasad AS. Zinc: mechanisms of host defense. J Nutr 2007;137(5):1345–9.
23. Maes M. Coenzyme Q10 deficiency in myalgic encephalomyelitis/chronic fatigue syndrome (ME/CFS) is related to fatigue, autonomic and neurocognitive symptoms and is another risk factor explaining the early mortality in ME/CFS due to cardiovascular disorder. Neuro Endocrinol Lett 2009;30(4):470–6.
24. Morris G, Anderson G, Berk M, Maes M. Coenzyme Q10 Depletion in Medical and Neuropsychiatric Disorders: Potential Repercussions and Therapeutic Implications. Mol Neurobiol 201348(3):883–903.
25. Teitelbaum J, Jandrain J, McGrew R. Treatment of Chronic Fatigue Syndrome and Fibromyalgia with D–Ribose – an Open-Label, Multicenter Study. Open Pain Journal2012:5:32-37.
26. Teitelbaum J. The Fatigue and Fibromyalgia Solution. Penguin, New York 2013.
27. Teitelbaum J, Bird B, Greenfield RM, et al. Effective Treatment of Chronic Fatigue Syndrome and Fibromyalgia – a Randomized, Double-Blind, Placebo-Controlled Intent to Treat Study. Jo Chronic Fatigue Syndrome 2001:8(2);3-28.
28. Sommer SJ. Finding Hope - when facing serious disease. Inspiring Stories, Healing Insights and Health Research. Amazon.com 2017. Chapter 9 - Meaning:123-142.
29. Also available from www.drstevensommer.com

Chapter 5 Choice and Progress

1. Barton A. *Recovery from CFS – 50 personal stories.* Author House UK Ltd 2008.

Chapter 6 Reaching Out - Building Social Scaffolding

1. Palmer A. *The Art of Asking -How I Learned to Stop Worrying and Let People Help.* Grand Central Publishing 2014. *(Available in Print, e-book, audiobook).*
2. House JS, Landis KR, Umberson D. Social relationships and health. Science 1988;241(4865): –540–5.
3. Orth-Gomer K, Johnson J V, Social network interaction and mortality. A six-year follow-up study of a random sample of the Swedish population. Journal of Chronic Diseases 1987;40(10):949–57.
4. Berkman LA, Syme SL. Social networks, host resistance, and mortality: a nine-year follow-up study of Alameda County residents. American Journal of Epidemiology 1979;109:186–204.
5. Bentall RP, Powell P, Nye FJ, Edwards RH. Predictors of response to treatment for chronic fatigue syndrome. Br J Psychiatry 2002;181:248-252.
6. Friedberg F, Leung DW, Quick J. Do support groups help people with chronic fatigue syndrome and fibromyalgia? A comparison of active and inactive members. J Rheumatol. 2005 Dec;32(12):2416-20.

Chapter 7 Restorative Sleep – Reclaiming Nigh Nigh's

1. Josev EK, Jackson ML, Bei B, et al. *Sleep Quality in Adolescents With Chronic Fatigue Syndrome/Myalgic Encephalomyelitis (CFS/ME).* J Clin Sleep Med. *2017 Sep 15;13(9):1057-1066.*
2. Burton A R, Rahman K, Kadota Y, et al. Reduced heart rate variability predicts poor sleep quality in a case-control study of chronic fatigue syndrome. Exp Brain Res. 2010; 204: 71-78.
3. Jackson M L, Bruck D, Sleep abnormalities in chronic fatigue syndrome/myalgic encephalomyelitis: a review. J Clin Sleep Med. 2012; 8: 719-728.
4. Van Cauwenbergh D, Nijs J, Kos D, et al. Malfunctioning of the autonomic nervous system in patients with chronic fatigue syndrome: a systematic literature review.
5. Eur J Clin Invest. 2014; 44: 516-526.
6. Orjatsalo M, Alakuijala A, Partinen M. Autonomic nervous system functioning related to nocturnal sleep in patients with chronic fatigue syndrome compared to tired controls. J Clin Sleep Med. 2018; 14: 163-171.
7. https://www.medscape.com/answers/1140322-124424/what-are-eeg-waveform-features-of-rapid-eye-movement-rem-sleep
8. https://www.anzacdental.com.au/images/Dr-Steven-Lin---the-five-stages-of-sleep-
9. Van Hoof E, De Becker P, Lapp C, et al. Defining the occurrence and influence of alpha-delta sleep in chronic fatigue syndrome. Am J Med Sci. 2007;333(2):78-84.
10. Milrad SF, Hall DL, Jutagir DR, et al. Poor sleep quality is associated with greater circulating pro-inflammatory cytokines and severity and frequency of chronic fatigue syndrome/myalgic encephalomyelitis (CFS/ME) symptoms in women. J Neuroimmunol. 2017 Feb 15;303:43-50.
11. Dr. Merrill Mitler, a sleep expert and neuroscientist https://newsinhealth.nih.gov/2013/04/benefits-slumber

12. Thorpy MJ ed. American Sleep Disorders Association. The International Classification of Sleep Disorders: Diagnosis and Coding Manual. Lawrence, Kansas: Allen Press. 1990.
13. Pajediene E, Bileviciute-Ljungar I, Friberg D. Sleep patterns among patients with chronic fatigue: A polysomnography-based study. Clin Respir J. 2018 Apr;12(4):1389-1397.
14. Ibid
15. Personal communication from Dr Daniel Lewis who has found the Oura ring very helpful for people with ME/CFS.
16. https://www.alexfergus.com/blog/oura-ring-review-new-smart-ring-continues-to-impress
17. Kupfer DJ, Spiker DG, Coble P, et al. Amitriptyline and EEG Sleep in Depressed patients: I. Drug Effect. Sleep, 1(2): 149-159.
18. Pagel JF, Parnes BL. Medications for the Treatment of Sleep Disorders: An Overview. Prim Care Companion J Clin Psychiatry. 2001; 3(3): 118–125.
19. Bested AC, Marshall LM. Review of Myalgic Encephalomyelitis/Chronic Fatigue Syndrome: an evidence-based approach to diagnosis and management by clinicians. Rev Environ Health. 2015;30(4):237. doi: 10.1515/reveh-2015-0026.

Chapter 8 Nutritional Wisdom

1. http://www.medicalsciencenavigator.com/physiology-of-self-renewal *(accessed September 2020)*
2. Campagnolo N, Johnston S, Collatz A, et al. Dietary and nutrition interventions for the therapeutic treatment of chronic fatigue syndrome/myalgic encephalomyelitis: a systematic review. J Hum Nutr Diet. 2017 Jun;30(3):247-259. doi: 10.1111/jhn.12435. Epub 2017 Jan 22.
3. Johnston SC, Staines DR, Marshall-Gradisnik SM. Epidemiological characteristics of chronic fatigue syndrome/myalgic encephalomyelitis in Australian patients. Clin Epidemiol 2016;8;97.
4. Raubenheimer D, Simpson S. Eat Like The Animals. Harper Collins 2020.
5. Shammas M A. Telomeres, lifestyle, cancer, and aging. Current opinion in clinical nutrition and metabolic care 2011, 14(1), 28–34.
6. Sommer SJ. Finding Hope -when facing serious disease. Inspiring Stories, Healing Insights and Health Research Amazon 2017;79-90.
7. Robbins J. Still Healthy at 100. Hodder & Stoughton 2006.
8. Smith-Spangler C, Brandea M, Hunter G, et al., Are organic foods safer or healthier than conventional alternatives? A systematic review. Annals of Internal Medicine 2012;157:348-66.
9. Brandt K, Leifert C, Sanderson R et al., Agroecosystem Management and Nutritional Quality of Plant Foods: The case of organic fruits and vegetables. Critical Reviews in Plant Sciences 2011; 30:1-2, 177-97.
10. Ibid. 27.
11. Lockie S, Lyons K, Lawrence G, et al., Choosing Organics: a path analysis of factors underlying the selection of organic food among Australian consumers. Appetite 2004; 43:135-46.
12. Lu C, Toepel K, Irish R, et al., Organic diets significantly lower children's dietary exposure to organophosphorus pesticides. Environmental Health Perspectives 2006; 114:260-63.

13. http://www.aap.org/en-us/about-the-aap/aap-press-room/Pages/American-Academy-of-Pediatrics-Weighs-In-For-the-First-Time-on-Organic-Foods-for-Children.aspx (accessed September 2020)
14. Lourie B and Smith R, Toxin Toxout: Getting harmful chemicals out of our bodies and our world. University of Queensland Press 2013:74.
15. Zhang L, Rana I, Shaffer RM, et al. Exposure to glyphosate-based herbicides and risk for non-Hodgkin lymphoma: A meta-analysis and supporting evidence. Mutat Res Jul-Sep 2019;781:186-206.
16. Ascherio A, Schwarzschild. The epidemiology of Parkinson's disease: risk factors and prevention. Lancet Neurol. Review 2016 Nov;15(12):1257-1272.
17. http://www.grazetech.com.au/sites/default/files/BFJ%20Mayer_minerals_nutrients_0.pdf (accessed May 2020)
18. Campbell TC, Jacobson H. Whole - Rethinking the Science of Nutrition. Ben Bella books, Inc. 2013:151-3.
19. Ibid
20. Eberhardt MV, Lee CY, Liu RH. Antioxidant Activity of Fresh Apples. Nature June 22, 2000;405 (6789): 903-4.
21. Boyer J, Liu RH. Review: Apple Phytochemicals and Their Health Effects. Nutrition Journal 2004; (5). http://www.nutritionj.com/content/3/1/5.
22. Ibid 20

Chapter 9 A Low GI Diet and the Mini-fast

1. *https://www.monashfodmap.com/about-fodmap-and-ibs/*
2. Bloomfield HE, Kane R, Koeller E, et al. Benefits and Harms of the Mediterranean Diet Compared to Other Diets (Internet).Washington (DC): Department of Veterans Affairs (US); 2015 Nov. free text at http://www.ncbi.nlm.nih.gov/pubmed/27559560 (accessed September 2020)
3. Johnston SC, Staines DR, Marshall-Gradisnik SM. Epidemiological characteristics of chronic fatigue syndrome/myalgic encephalomyelitis in Australian patients. Clin Epidemiol 2016;8;97.
4. https://blog.rosemarycottageclinic.co.uk/2017/11/19/carbohydrates-not-animal-fats-linked-to-heart-disease-across-42-european-countries/?fbclid=IwAR32nbNwH6pqj5C0LrpZei6G9R-cFqmJCkXLWpH5nrZhx20u3QMFBuskxq4
5. Wahls T. The Wahls Protocol, Penguin New York 2014.Also see https://terrywahls.com/about-the-wahls-protocol/
6. Ibid
7. https://www.aboutibs.org/low-fodmap-diet/five-low-fodmap-diet-pitfalls-and-what-you-can-do-to-avoid-them
8. https://www.health.harvard.edu/diseases-and-conditions/glycemic-index-and-glycemic-load-for-100-foods
9. https://www.gisymbol.com/about-glycemic-index/
10. Fremont, Coomans D, Massart S, et al. High-throughput 16S rRNA gene sequencing reveals alterations of intestinal microbiota in myalgic encephalomyelitis/chronic fatigue syndrome patients. 2013 Aug; 22:50-6.
11. Biedermann L, Rogler G. The intestinal microbiota: its role in health and disease. Eur J Pediatr. 2015 Feb;174(2):151-67.
12. Brandt LJ. Fecal Microbiota Transplant: Respice, Adspice, Prospice. J Clin Gastroenterol. 2015 Nov-Dec;49 Suppl 1:S65-8.

13. Borody TJ, Nowak A, Torres M, et al. Bacteriotherapy in chronic fatigue syndrome: a retrospective review. Am J Gastroenterol. 2012;107(suppl 1):S591–S592.
14. Rao AV, Bested AC, Beaulne TM, et al. A randomized, double-blind, placebo-controlled pilot study of a probiotic in emotional symptoms of chronic fatigue syndrome. Gut Pathog. 2009 Mar 19;1(1):6. 1-6.
15. Holmqvist S, Chutna O, Bousset L, et al. Direct evidence of Parkinson pathology spread from the gastrointestinal tract to the brain in rats. Acta Neuropathol. 2014 Dec;128(6):805-20.
16. Liebert A, Bicknell B, Johnstone DM, et al. "Photobiomics": Can Light, Including Photobiomodulation, Alter the Microbiome? Photobiomodulation, Photomedicine, and Laser Surgery 2019;37(11):681–693.
17. Mischley LK, Lau RC, Bennett RD. Role of Diet and Nutritional Supplements in Parkinson's Disease Progression. Oxid Med Cell Longev. 2017;2017:6405278.
18. Torkova AA, Ksenia V, Lisitskaya V, et al. Physicochemical and functional properties of *Cucurbita maxima* pumpkin pectin and commercial citrus and apple pectins: A comparative evaluation. PLoS One. 2018; 13(9): e0204261.
19. Maes M, Leunis JC. Normalization of leaky gut in chronic fatigue syndrome (CFS) is accompanied by a clinical improvement: effects of age, duration of illness and the translocation of LPS from gram-negative bacteria. Neuro Endocrinol Lett 2008;29(6):902–10.
20. Patterson RE, Sears DD. Metabolic Effects of Intermittent Fasting. Annu Rev Nutr. 2017 Aug 21;37:371-393. doi: 10.1146/annurev-nutr-071816-064634. Epub 2017 Jul 17.
21. Horne BD, Muhlestein JB, Anderson JL. Health effects of intermittent fasting: hormesis or harm? A systematic review. Am J Clin Nutr. 2015 Aug;102(2):464-70. doi: 10.3945/ajcn.115.109553. Epub 2015 Jul 1.
22. https://www.healthline.com/nutrition/fasting-benefits#section1 [accessed May 2022]
23. Ibid

Further Reading on Diet

1. https://www.abc.net.au/radionational/programs/bigideas/dr-michael-mosley-on-how-to-eat-and-what-to-eat/11566528
2. https://thefast800.com/?gclid=EAIaIQobChMImryL8quT5QIVVx0rCh2r0wQ4EAAYASAAEgKiBPD_BwE
3. Christian Allen PhD, Wolfgang Lutz MD. Life Without Bread - How a Low Carbohydrate Diet Can Save Your Life, McGraw Hill Professional 2000.
4. https://terrywahls.com/about-the-wahls-protocol/
5. https://www.phoenixhelix.com/
6. Dr Pimentel is a US gastroenterologist and leading researcher in the field of IBS and SIBO. GOOGLE him for interviews.
7. https://www.ncbi.nlm.nih.gov/pubmed/29372991
8. https://www.ncbi.nlm.nih.gov/pubmed/14992438

Chapter 10 Pacing and Energy Envelope Theory

1. *Van der Werf SP, Prins JB, Vercoulen JH, et al. Identifying physical activity patterns in Chronic Fatigue Syndrome using actigraphic assessment. J Psychosom Res 2000;49(5)373-79.*

2. Houdenhouve B, Neerinkx B, Onghena P, et al., Premorbid "overactive" lifestyle in Chronic fatigue Syndrome and Fibromyalgia an etiological factor or proof of good citizenship? J Psychosom Res 2001;51(4):571-76.
3. Nijs J, Van Eupen I, Vandecouter J, et al., Can Pacing self-management modify physical behavior and symptom severity in Chronic Fatigue Syndrome? A case series. JRRD 2009;46(7): 985–996.
4. Jason L, Melrose H, Lerman A, Burroughs V, Lewis K, King C, Frankenberry E. Managing chronic fatigue syndrome: Overview and case study. AAOHN J 1999;47:17–21.
5. Jason LA, Brown M, Brown A, Energy Conservation/Envelope Theory Interventions to Help Patients with Myalgic Encephalomyelitis/Chronic Fatigue Syndrome. Fatigue. 2013 Jan 14;1(1-2):27-42. Epub 2012 Aug 8.
6. Jason LA, Benton M. The impact of energy modulation on physical functioning and fatigue and severity among patients with ME/CFS. Patient Educ Couns 2009;77(2):237–41.
7. Goudsmit, EM. The psychological aspects and management of chronic fatigue syndrome[PhD thesis]. Brunel University, UK; London: 1996. Available on the Internet from Ethos: http:// ethos.bl.uk/Home.do
8. Goudsmit EM, Nijs J, Jason LA, Wallman KE. Pacing as a strategy to improve energy management in myalgic encephalomyelitis/chronic fatigue syndrome: a consensus document. Disability and Rehabilitation. 2011.
9. Goudsmit EM, Howes S. Pacing: A strategy to improve energy management in chronic fatigue syndrome. Health Psychology Update. 2008; 17(1):46–52.
10. Goudsmit EM, Ho-Yen DO, Dancey CP. Learning to cope with chronic illness. Efficacy of a multi-component treatment for people with chronic fatigue syndrome. Patient Education and Counseling. 2009; 77:231–36
11. Hayes SC, Luoma J, Bond F, Masuda A, Lillis J. Acceptance and Commitment Therapy: Model, processes, and outcomes. Behavior Research and Therapy. 2006;44(1):1–25.
12. Ibid,10.

Chapter 11 Micro-Rehab

1. *Lien K, Johansen B,* Marit B. Veierød, *et al. Abnormal blood lactate accumulation during repeated exercise testing in myalgic encephalomyelitis/chronic fatigue syndrome. Physiology Reports Open Access 2019;7(11).*
2. Morris G, Maes M. Mitochondrial dysfunctions in myalgic encephalomyelitis/chronic fatigue syndrome explained by activated immuno-inflammatory, oxidative and nitrosative stress pathways. Metab Brain Dis. 2014 Mar;29(1):19-36
3. Nijs J, Nees A, Paul L, et al., Altered immune response to exercise in patients with chronic fatigue syndrome/myalgic encephalomyelitis: a systematic literature review. Exerc Immunol Rev. 2014;20:94-116.
4. White AT, Light AR, Hughen RW, Bateman L, Thomas B, et al. Severity of symptom flare after moderate exercise is linked to cytokine activity in chronic fatigue syndrome. Psychophysiology 2010;47(4):615–24.
5. Montoya JG, Holmes TH, Anderson JN, et al. Cytokine signature associated with disease severity in chronic fatigue syndrome patients. Proc Natl Acad Sci U S A July 31, 2017; doi: 10.1073/pnas.1710519114

6. Beyond Myalgic Encephalomyelitis/Chronic Fatigue Syndrome: Redefining an Illness. Committee on the Diagnostic Criteria for Myalgic Encephalomyelitis/Chronic Fatigue Syndrome; Board on the Health of Select Populations; Institute of Medicine. Source Washington (DC): National Academies Press (US); 2015 Feb. The National Academies Collection: Reports funded by National Institutes of Health.
7. Ibid 3
8. https://www.who.int/news-room/fact-sheets/detail/rehabilitation
9. tps://dictionary.cambridge.org/dictionary/english/exercise
10. Pedersen BK, Saltin B. Exercise as medicine - evidence for prescribing exercise as therapy in 26 different chronic diseases. Scand J Med Sci Sports. 2015 Dec;25 Suppl 3:1-72. doi: 10.1111/sms.12581. Review.
11. Boushel R, Lundby C, Qvortrup K, et al. Mitochondrial Plasticity With Exercise Training and Extreme Environments. Exerc Sport Sci Rev. 2014 Jul 24.
12. Morris G, Maes M. Mitochondrial dysfunctions in myalgic encephalomyelitis/chronic fatigue syndrome explained by activated immuno-inflammatory, oxidative and nitrosative stress pathways. Metab Brain Dis. 2014 Mar;29(1):19-36.
13. Pardaens K, Haagdorens L, Van Wambeke P, et al., How relevant are exercise capacity measures for evaluating treatment effects in chronic fatigue syndrome? Results from a prospective, multidisciplinary outcome study. Clin Rehabil. 2006; 20(1):56-66.
14. ME/CFS The biomedical basis, diagnosis, treatment and management. International Research Symposium Geelong Australia, March 12-15.
15. https://vimeo.com/ondemand/klimasexercise
16. http://recoveryfromcfs.org/ch11/
17. http://cfsrecoveryproject.com/how-to-benefit-from-exercise-even-if-you-have-chronic-fatigue-syndrome/
18. Ibid
19. Ibid 15
20. Marchant J. Cure. Text publishing Melbourne 2016;82-90.
21. http://www.theguardian.com/society/2016/feb/15/it-was-like-being-buried-alive-victim-of-chronic-fatigue-syndrome

Chapter 12 Preparation for Exercise

1. http://www.cdc.gov/physicalactivity/basics/measuring/exertion.htm (*Note: The original Borg RPE Scale is 6 to 20*)
2. Bested AC, Marshall LM. Review of Myalgic Encephalomyelitis/Chronic Fatigue Syndrome: an evidence-based approach to diagnosis and management by clinicians. Rev Environ Health. 2015;30(4):238. doi: 10.1515/reveh-2015-0026.
3. http://www.cdc.gov/physicalactivity/basics/measuring/exertion.htm
4. https://www.painscience.com/articles/delayed-onset-muscle-soreness.php
5. https://health.clevelandclinic.org/ok-push-pain-exercise/?utm_source=marketo&utm_medium=email&utm_campaign=health+essentials+daily+tip+10-05-18&utmcontent=story1+cta&mkt_tok=eyJpIjoiT1dRNVltWm1OamRsTXpRdyIsInQiOiJIRHI1dVZHU2pNaW9WZ Dg0YkQ3aFRheFViUnh1ZERGZ lwvU3ZFc1wvYjhWb0hwNTV1aUFENGsrZ0xJVElLdFpjWnZV UWxFcTgrV1I5Z0VkZmQydOM2bU96dE4yTUN1dlJJVTlw QjBPK0I0WitndGZSSdlN0U0RMbEdPOGR6bUJ2ajFENm0%3D

6. Christina B. Dillon, CB, Perry IJ. Does replacing sedentary behaviour with light or moderate to vigorous physical activity modulate inflammatory status in adults? Int J Behav Nutr Phys Act. 2017; 14: 138.
7. Gerwyn M , Maes M. Mechanisms Explaining Muscle Fatigue and Muscle Pain in Patients with Myalgic Encephalomyelitis/Chronic Fatigue Syndrome (ME/CFS): a Review of Recent Findings 2017. Curr Rheumatol Rep. Jan;19(1):1.
8. Lynch A, Blucher P. Taking Nothing For Granted. A sportsman's fight against Chronic Fatigue. Harper Collins 2005. E6:11. EBook available from Harper.
9. Vallings R Chronic Fatigue Syndrome ME - Symptom, Diagnosis, Management. Calico Publishing 2012, Auckland.
10. Ibid 8
11. Buijze GA, Sierevelt IN, van der Heijden BCJM, et al. The Effect of **Cold** Showering on Health and Work: A Randomized Controlled Trial. PLoS One. 2016; 11(9): e0161749.

Chapter 13 STOP! The Rest Activity Dance

1. Benson H, *The Relaxation Response: HarperCollins 1975.*
2. Sommer SJ. Finding Hope - when facing serious disease. Inspiring Stories, Healing Insights and Health Research. Amazon.com 2017;67-95. Also available from www.drstevensommer.com

Chapter 14 GO...gently! The Rest Activity Dance

1. *http://cfsrecoveryproject.com/how-to-benefit-from-exercise-even-if-you-have-chronic-fatigue-syndrome/*
2. Pedersen BK, Saltin B. Exercise as medicine - evidence for prescribing exercise as therapy in 26 different chronic diseases. Scand J Med Sci Sports. 2015 Dec;25 Suppl 3:1-72. doi: 10.1111/sms.12581. Review.
3. Boushel R, Lundby C, Qvortrup K, et al. Mitochondrial Plasticity With Exercise Training and Extreme Environments. Exerc Sport Sci Rev. 2014 Jul 24.
4. Gordon B, Lubitz L, Promising outcomes of an adolescent chronic fatigue syndrome inpatient programme. J Paediatr Child Health. 2009 May;45(5):286-90.
5. http://www.theage.com.au/national/inpatient-program-swamped-by-children-with-chronic-fatigue-20100206-njy1.html [Accessed March 2016]
6. http://shepherdworks.com.au/disease-information/low-fodmap-diet *(accessed March 2019)*
7. http://www.austin.org.au/Adult_CFS *[accessed July 2019]*
8. Ciccone DS, Chandler HK, Natelson BH. Illness trajectories in the chronic fatigue syndrome: a longitudinal study of improvers versus non-improvers. J Nerv Ment Dis 2010;198(7):486–93.
9. Pheby D, Saffron L. Risk factors for severe ME/CFS. Biol Med 2009;1(4):50–74.
10. Bell DS. Twenty-five year follow-up in chronic fatigue syndrome: Rising Incapacity. Mass CFIDS Assoc. Continuing Education Lecture April 16, 2011.

Chapter 15 Defuse the Loop

1. *Sommer SJ. Mind-body medicine and holistic approaches: the scientific evidence. Australian Family Physician 1996;25(8):1233–1244.*
2. Rosenkranz MA, Davidson RJ, Maccoon DG, et al. A comparison of mindfulness-based stress reduction and an active control in modulation of neurogenic

inflammation. Behav Immun. 2013 Jan;27(1):174-84. doi: 10.1016/j.bbi.2012.10.013. Epub 2012 Oct 22. PMID: 23092711 Free PMC article. Clinical Trial

3. Pascoe MC, Thompson DR, Jenkins ZM, et al. Mindfulness mediates the physiological markers of stress: Systematic review and meta-analysis. J Psychiatr Res. 2017 Dec;95:156-178. Review.
4. Eva-Britt Hysing, Lena Smith, Måns Thulin, et al. Detection of systemic inflammation in severely impaired chronic pain patients and effects of a multimodal pain rehabilitation program Scand J Pain 2019 Apr 24;19(2):235-244.
5. Doidge N. The Brain That Changes Itself: Stories of Personal Triumph from the Frontiers of Brain Science. Viking Press 2007.
6. Mayo K R, Support from neurobiology for spiritual techniques for anxiety: a brief review. J Health Care Chaplain. 2009;16(1-2):53-7.
7. Sommer SJ. Finding Hope - when facing serious disease. Inspiring Stories, Healing Insights and Health Research. Chapter 8 Mind Body Weaving. Amazon.com 2017:107-122. Also available from www.drstevensommer.com
8. Ong W, Stohler C, Herr D. Role of the Prefrontal Cortex in Pain Processing Mol Neurobiol . 2019 Feb;56(2):1137-1166. doi: 10.1007/s12035-018-1130-9. Epub 2018 Jun 6.
9. Zalcman S, Savina I, Wise RA. Interleukin-6 increases sensitivity to the locomotor-stimulating effects of amphetamine in rats. Brain Res 1999;847:276–83.
10. Saal D, Dong Y, Bonci A, Malenka R. Drugs of abuse and stress trigger a common synaptic adaption in dopamine neurons. Neuron 2003;37(4):577–82.
11. Gellhorn E. The emotions and the ergotropic and trophotropic systems. Psychologische Forschung 1970;34:48–94.
12. Miller GE, Cohen S. Psychological interventions and the immune system: A meta-analytic review and critique. Health Psych 2001;20:47–63.
13. https://www.healthrising.org/blog/2020/11/13/nice-discards-graded-exercise-therapy-cbt-treatment-chronic-fatigue-syndrome/
14. https://www.cochrane.org/CD001027/DEPRESSN_cognitive-behaviour-therapy-chronic-fatigue-syndrome
15. Price JR, Mitchell E, Tidy E, Hunot V. Cognitive behaviour therapy for chronic fatigue syndrome in adults. Cochrane Database Syst Rev. 2008;(3):CD001027.
16. Gupta A. Unconscious amygdala fear conditioning in a subset of chronic fatigue syndrome patients. Medical Hypotheses. 2002; 59:727–735.
17. http://www.guptaprogramme.com [accessed March 2020]
18. http://www.mickeltherapy.com/ [accessed March 2020]
19. https://juliacameronlive.com/basic-tools/morning-pages/
20. Neff K, Self Compassion. Hodder and Stoughton 2011.
21. Germer CK, The Mindful Path to Self-compassion -freeing yourself from destructive thoughts and emotions. Guilford Press New York 2009.

Chapter 16 Healing Notes - Ruth's Story circa 2021

Summing Up

1. *McIntyre A. Chronic Fatigue Syndrome – a practical guide. Thorsons London 1998:1-33.*
2. Vallings R. The Pocket Guide to Chronic Fatigue Syndrome ME – Key Facts and Tips for Improved Health. Calico Publishing 2017, Auckland:16,17.

Future Research

1. *Arbesman S, The Half-Life of Facts: Why Everything We Know Has an Expiration Date. Penguin Group USA 2012.*
2. Hadgkiss EJ, Jelinek GA, Weiland TJ et al. Health-related quality of life outcomes at 1 and 5 years after a residential retreat promoting lifestyle modification for people with multiple sclerosis, Neurol Sci. 2013 Feb;34(2):187-95.
3. Liebert A, Bicknell B, Johnstone DM, et al. "Photobiomics": Can Light, Including Photobiomodulation, Alter the Microbiome? Photobiomodulation, Photomedicine, and Laser Surgery 2019;37(11):681–693.
4. Cabanas H, Muraki K, Staines D, et al. Naltrexone Restores Impaired Transient Receptor Potential Melastatin 3 Ion Channel Function in Natural Killer Cells From Myalgic Encephalomyelitis/Chronic Fatigue Syndrome Patients Front Immunol. 2019 Oct 31;10:2545.
5. Patten DK, Schultz BG, Berlau DJ. The Safety and Efficacy of Low-Dose Naltrexone in the Management of Chronic Pain and Inflammation in Multiple Sclerosis, Fibromyalgia, Crohn's Disease, and Other Chronic Pain Disorders. Pharmacotherapy. 2018 Mar;38(3):382-389. Review.
6. Metyas S, Chen CL, Yeter K, et al. Low Dose Naltrexone in the Treatment of Fibromyalgia. Curr Rheumatol Rev. 2018;14(2):177-180.
7. Toljan K, Vrooman B. Low-Dose Naltrexone (LDN)-Review of Therapeutic Utilization. Med Sci (Basel). 2018 Sep 21;6(4):82.
8. Chakravarthy K, Chaudhry H, Williams K, et al. Review of the Uses of Vagal Nerve Stimulation in Chronic Pain Management. Curr Pain Headache Rep. 2015 Dec;19(12):54.
9. Paccione CE, Diep LM, Stubhaug A, Jacobsen HB. Motivational nondirective resonance breathing versus transcutaneous vagus nerve stimulation in the treatment of fibromyalgia: study protocol for a randomized controlled trial. Trials. 2020 Sep 23;21(1):808.
10. Conde-Antón A, Hernando-Garijo I, Jiménez-Del-Barrio S, et al. Effects of transcranial direct current stimulation and transcranial magnetic stimulation in patients with fibromyalgia. A systematic review Neurologia (Engl Ed) 2020 Oct 15;S0213-4853(20)30278-4.

ABOUT THE AUTHORS

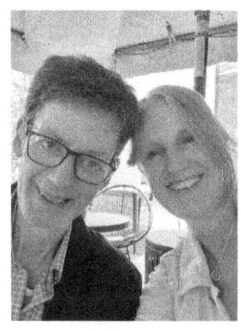

Steven Sommer M.B.,B.S FRACGP

Steven graduated from Monash University Medical School in 1984. He then worked in hospital settings over 4 years, before successfully completing his general practice training to become a Fellow of the Royal Australian College of General Practitioners in 1991.

He developed a special interest in mindfulness-based stress management in the early 90's whilst working as a GP and senior lecturer at Monash University's Department of General Practice and he was an invited Grand Round presenter on this topic at several major teaching hospitals.

In 1993 he took on the role of president of the Whole Health Institute of Australasia (WHI); a non-profit educational organisation. In 1996 his health collapsed; he was eventually diagnosed with ME/CFS and too unwell to continue, he had to relinquish all his previous roles.

It took 11 years, but by 2007 he'd found a way to restore enough from ME/CFS to return to general practice and teaching at Deakin University Medical School. However, further health crises in 2011, unrelated to ME/CFS, left him unable to continue as a practitioner. This has opened a space for him to research and share his ideas and insights through his writing. This is the first of two books he's authored on ME/CFS. (*ME/CFS – A Path Back to Life* will be released shortly.)

His first book, Finding Hope (2017), was well-received. (see wwwdrstevensommer.com).

In 2019 Steven was invited to join the inaugural Medical Advisory Committee for Emerge (ME/CFS) Australia.

Tori Sommer B.App.Sc.(Chiro), BA(psych).

After completing her BA(psych) at Melbourne University, Tori worked and travelled through Europe for 2 years before returning to five more years of study at the Royal Melbourne Institute of technology (RMIT) to become a chiropractor. During her chiropractic studies she joined the Whole Health Institute (WHI) and headed up the student committee. Her interest in performing and singing led her to meeting Steven. They met on stage as part of the WHI comedy troupe performing at a student healthcare conference in 1991.

Tori worked and ran her own clinic as a chiropractor until 2011 when her energies were needed to care full time for Steven. Over these difficult years she has found solace in exploring her interests and developing her skills in the Arts, including children's book illustration. She has a been accepted to complete an honors degree in Visual Arts at Deakin University in Geelong.

Steven and Tori recently celebrated 25 years of marriage. They live in Geelong together with their three cats, Old Man Claude, Princess Pippy (Pip) and Tooley Scrumptious (Scrumps).

ABOUT THE AUTHORS

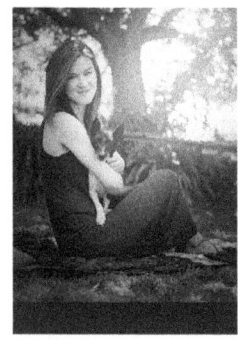

Ruth Gador

Ruth lives in Geelong with her family and dog Buddy!

She enjoys going for walks in nature, the ocean, reading, writing and playing music. She is currently teaching violin to students and loves sharing her joy of music with them.

One of her interests includes health and healing and she enjoys the benefits of sound therapy, and in particular listening to sound bowls.

GLOSSARY OF ACRONYMS

ADLS	Activities of Daily Living
ANTS	Automatic Negative Thoughts
CPET	Cardiopulmonary Testing
CI	Chronotropic Intolerance
CFS	Chronic Fatigue Syndrome
CFIDS	Chronic Fatigue Immune Deficiency Syndrome
CBT	Cognitive Behavioural Therapy
DOMS	Delayed Onset Muscle Soreness
EEG	Electroencephalogram
FODMAP	Fermentable Oligo-, Di-, Mono-saccharides And Polyols
fMRI	Functional Magnetic Resonance Imaging
GET	Graded Exercise Therapy
NMH	Neurally Mediated Hypotension
HR	Heart rate
MMC	Migrating Motor Complex
ME	Myalgic Encephalomyelitis
MS	Multiple Sclerosis
NMH	Neurally Mediated Hypotension
OI	Orthostatic Intolerance
PD	Parkinson's Disease
PEM	Post-exertional malaise

PETS	Positive Emotional Thoughts
PSG	Polysomnography
POTS	Postural Orthostatic Tachycardia Syndrome
PTSD	Post Traumatic Stress Disorder
RPE	Rating of Perceived Exertion (1 to 10)
RR	Relaxation Response
RMHR	Resting Morning Heart Rate
SEID	Systemic Exertion Intolerance Disease
SWAT	Special Weapons and Tactical

Lightning Source UK Ltd.
Milton Keynes UK
UKHW012209061022
410049UK00001B/83

9 780995 434554